Pocket

Regional
and Clinical
Anatomy

Peter H Abrahams MB, BS

Senior Lecturer in Anatomy
The Middlesex Hospital Medical School
University of London

Examiner in Anatomy to
The Royal College of Surgeons of England
—Primary FRCS Examination

Matthew J Thatcher MB, BS, FRCS, FRCS(ED)

Registrar in Diagnostic Radiology
Royal Free Hospital, London

Churchill Livingstone

Edinburgh London Melbourne and New York 1986

CHURCHILL LIVINGSTONE
Medical Division of Longman Group Limited

Distributed in the United States of America by
Churchill Livingstone Inc., 1560 Broadway, New York,
N.Y. 10036, and by associated companies, branches
and representatives throughout the world

First published 1981 (Pitman Publishing Ltd)
   Reprinted 1984
   Reprinted 1986 (Churchill Livingstone)

ISBN 0 443 03651 9

British Library Cataloguing in Publication Data
Abrahams, Peter H.
   Pocket examiner in regional and
   clinical anatomy.
   1. Anatomy, Surgical and topographical
   I. Title
   611'9   QM531

Library of Congress Cataloging in Publication Data

Printed at The Bath Press, Avon

Contents

Preface

Examinations and assessments are necessary evils for students and teachers alike. None causes more anxiety than the oral, or viva, examination when, often for the first time, examiner and candidate meet face to face. Preparing for both oral and written examinations in anatomy is a long process, there being no short cuts to learning the facts.

However, having analysed both written and oral undergraduate examinations over some years, we have found a constant core of questions turning up in all medical schools. These tend to fall into one of two categories, in the same pattern as presented in this book: first, the information question involving simple factual recall and, second, the applied questions, often involving a higher level of comprehension and some-times a little digression from pure gross anatomy into the fields of embryology, radiology, surgery and medicine. This type of applied question tends to turn up more frequently in oral examinations. It is ex-tremely difficult to prepare for any oral examination except by question and answer practice, which we hope this book will stimulate, especially amongst small tutorial groups of students.

This book is intended to supplement and not to replace the standard texts on anatomy, and for this reason every question is referenced to a suitable section or illustration from one of the better known anatomy textbooks.

We sincerely hope that this little book will stimu-late discussion between students, as nothing is more soul-destroying, particularly in anatomy, than sitting alone trying to amass the facts. We also hope that our efforts will make the anatomy viva a little less daunting.

PHA
MJT

Acknowledgements

We would like to thank all the students and colleagues who encouraged us to put these short questions and answers into a book format. Our special thanks go to Professor I. Glazer and Professor G. Gitlin, whose constructive criticism helped to consolidate our initial ideas during the participation of a WHO medical education project at Beer-Sheva, Israel. This contribution was made possible by the continuous support of Dr A. H. Taba, Director of the Eastern Mediterranean Regional Office of the WHO, to whom we extend our gratitude. We would also like to thank Mr J. Walker, BSc, for his biographical notes in the back of the volume, and for his help in proof reading.

To Miss Elisabeth Smale and Miss Anne Danagher go our special thanks for their patience in deciphering our awful writing and typing the manuscript.

1
Key to references and further reading

A *Gray's Anatomy*, Warwick, R. and Williams, P. L., 35th British edn. (Longman, Edinburgh, 1973)

B *Anatomy—A Regional Study of Human Structure*, Gardner, E., Gray, D. J. and O'Rahilly, R., 4th edn. (W. B. Saunders, Philadelphia, 1975)

C *Textbook of Anatomy*, Hollinshead, W. H., 3rd edn. (Harper and Row, Hagerston, Maryland, 1974)

D *Clinical Anatomy. A Revision and Applied Anatomy for Clinical Students*, Ellis, H., 6th edn. (Blackwell Scientific Publications, Oxford, 1977)

E *Clinical Anatomy for Medical Students*, Snell, R. S. (Little, Brown and Company, Boston, 1973)

F *Grant's Method of Anatomy*, Basmajian, J. V., 9th edn. (Williams & Wilkins, Baltimore, 1975)

G *Grant's Atlas of Anatomy*, Anderson, J. E., 7th edn. (Williams & Wilkins, Baltimore, 1978)

H *A Colour Atlas of Human Anatomy*, McMinn, R. M. H. and Hutchings, R. T. (Wolfe Medical Books, London, 1977)

I *An Atlas of Anatomy Basic to Radiology*, Meschan, I. (W. B. Saunders, Philadelphia, 1975)

J *An Atlas of Radiological Anatomy*, Weir, J. and Abrahams, P. H. (Pitman Medical, Tunbridge Wells, 1978)

2
Questions

HEAD AND NECK

A Bones of the skull

Information questions

1 Which skull bones form in membrane?

2 Which parts of the temporal bone develop in cartilage?

3 What is the metopic suture of the frontal bone?

4 What are the vertex, inion, glabella and crista galli?

5 The spine of the sphenoid has most important relations. What structures does this bony point protect?

6 Describe the foramina of the sphenoid bone. Which structures pass through them?

7 Where would you find the diploic veins?

8 What are emissary veins?

9 The conchae of the nose are formed by which bones?

10 Where is the foramen lacerum on a skull? Describe its relationship to the carotid artery.

11 What is the 'antrum' in the facial skeleton?

12 What class and type of joint is the basi-occipital/basisphenoid joint and when does it normally fuse?

Applied questions

13 How is the neonatal skull different from that of the adult?

14 What consequences during parturition do you think may result from the relative small size of the fetal mastoid process?

15 A full sailor's beard overlies which bones?

16 A fracture in the region of the pterion may have serious consequences. What structure is at greatest risk in this injury?

17 What have the mastoid, ethmoid, sphenoid and maxilla in common?

18 Why might direct trauma and fracture of the hyoid bone prove dangerous?

19 Why might a fracture of the lower mandible cause numbness of the lower lip?

B Cranial fossae
   Cranial meninges
   Dural venous sinuses

Information questions

20 Where on a skull would you define the borders of the anterior and middle cranial fossae?

21 What structure lies between the clinoid processes?

22 What is the clivus, and which portion of the brain lies against it?

23 Which structures emerge from the skull through the jugular foramen?

24 Describe the relationship of the XIIth cranial nerve to the carotid arteries.

25 Where might you find the arachnoid granulations and lacunae within the skull?

26 What are the falces? Describe their functions.

27 Describe the contents of the cavernous sinus.

28 Which vessels drain into the cavernous sinus?

29 How would you find the superior sagittal sinus in a 6-month-old baby?

30 What vessels drain into the straight sinus?

31 Describe the walls of the superior sagittal sinus.

Applied questions

32 A patient presents with an increase in hat and glove size, and it is suggested that he may have a pituitary tumour. Which plain x-ray do you think might confirm this diagnosis?

33 A small depressed fracture of the vertex may cause thrombosis of the superior sagittal sinus. Why might this rapidly cause unconsciousness due to increased intracranial pressure?

34 On a slit Towne's x-ray of the skull you should see the arcuate eminence of the temporal bone. What important structure causes this prominence?

35 A fracture through the pterygoid canal might damage which nerve fibres and with what consequences?

36 What is an important function of the tegmen tympani?

37 Why might a fractured cribriform plate of the ethmoid bone lead to a loss of smell (anosmia) and a runny nose (rhinorrhea)?

38 By which route might you aspirate a subdural haematoma from a small baby?

39 Why might pressing a boil on the cheek lead to a VIth nerve palsy?

40 Using x-rays, how can one view the major dural venous sinuses?

C Face
   Scalp
   Parotid region

Information questions

41 What have the platsyma and the dartos muscle in common?

42 What is the sensory nerve supply to the skin over the angle of the jaw?

43 What is the sensory supply to the area of the upper lip covered by a moustache?

44 Describe the sphincter muscles of the face and their innervation.

45 What are the scalp's five layers?

46 Describe the arteries that anastomose in the scalp. From where do they originate?

47 Describe the secretomotor pathway to the parotid gland.

48 What arteries, veins and nerves lie within the parotid gland?

Applied questions

49 What are the effects on lacrimation of a damaged orbicularis oculi?

50 Describe the area affected by herpes zoster in the area supplied by the maxillary division of the trigeminal nerve.

51 Which are the most important muscles of facial expression?

52 How will the vestibule of the mouth be affected by a damaged VIIth cranial nerve?

53 Why might a lesion of the ophthalmic division of the trigeminal nerve be dangerous to the eye?

54 Where would a collection of blood or pus lie within the five layers of the scalp?

55 A young man with long flowing locks leans over his lathe and catches his hair in the machinery. Along which layer is he likely to be 'scalped'?

56 A generalised scalp infection will drain to which groups of lymph nodes?

57 How may an abscess on the scalp endanger the brain?

58 Why is mumps so painful?

59 Why might cancer of the parotid gland present clinically as a facial paralysis?

60 If the auriculotemporal nerve is cut some distance beyond its origin, what will happen to the parotid gland?

61 Where would you look to find the opening of the parotid duct, and how might you palpate this duct on the face?

D Temporal and infratemporal regions Temporomandibular joint

Information questions

62 In dissection, you often find the middle meningeal artery encircled by a small nerve. Which is it?

63 What fibres does the nerve of the pterygoid canal (Vidian nerve) carry?

64 Describe the origin and course of the middle meningeal artery.

65 Which muscle protrudes and opens the jaw?

66 What is unusual about the structure of the temporomandibular joint?

67 Describe the movements of the temporomandibular joint.

68 What structures attach to or hook round the hamulus?

69   What structures attach to the pterygomandibu-
     lar raphe?

Applied questions

70   To stop an extradural haemorrhage, which
     artery would you wish to tie and through
     which foramen does it enter the skull?

71   Why might an infection deep in the pterygoid
     region be of danger to the eye?

72   Why do babies who have a forceps delivery
     more commonly present with temporary facial
     palsies?

73   On clenching the jaw tight, what structure can
     you palpate lying on the contracted masseter?

74   Where does the dentist inject an anaesthetic if
     he wishes to numb your lower teeth?

75   Why is the sphenopalatine ganglion sometimes
     called the ganglion of 'hay fever'?

76   If you wished to visualise the articular tubercle,
     tympanic plate and external auditory meatus,
     what x-ray would you order?

77   Why might a dislocation of the temporomandi-
     bular joint occur during a boring anatomy lec-
     ture?

78   What muscles may be involved in trismus?

**E   Orbit
     Eyeball**

Information questions

79   Which bones form the orbit?

80   Which nerves pass through the superior and
     inferior orbital fissures, respectively?

81   Describe the fascial sheath of the eyeball
     (Tenon's capsule).

82 Which extraocular muscles originate from the tendinous ring?

83 What is the major refracting surface of the eye? Discuss its vascularity.

84 Name the six major extraocular muscles and their effects on the position of the eyeball.

85 Describe the muscles of the iris. What is their nerve supply?

86 Why is the optic nerve not a 'true' cranial nerve?

87 Where, on dissection, would you look for the ciliary ganglion?

88 Which fibres synapse in the ciliary ganglion?

89 What major differences are there between the long and short ciliary nerves?

Applied questions

90 What is the anatomical difference between a Meibomian cyst and a stye?

91 Explain two different causes of a drooped upper eyelid (ptosis).

92 What is the anatomical explanation of swelling of the optic disc (papilloedema)?

93 How do you test accommodation, and which nerve fibres are involved?

94 Why is blockage of the central artery of the retina a disaster?

95 A patient comes into your clinic with ptosis, a dilated pupil and an eyeball that looks down and laterally. What might you diagnose?

96 If a patient came to you with progressive ptosis of the right eye but with normal examination of cranial nerves III, IV and VI, why might a chest x-ray be advisable?

9

97 Where is the blind spot in a normal eye?

98 If you use a drug to dilate the pupil for ophthalmoscopy, why might you cause an attack of
raised intraocular pressure (acute glaucoma)?

99 A patient complains he cannot turn his right
eye to the right. What nerve lesion is the likely
cause?

F Nose
Paranasal air sinuses
Palate
Tonsil
Pharynx

Information questions

100 The nasal septum is formed from which structures?

101 Describe the functions of the nasal cavity and
also those attributed to the paranasal air
sinuses.

102 What opens into the lateral wall of the nasal
cavity?

103 Which arteries anastomose on the anteroinferior part of the nasal septum and from where do
they originate?

104 What is the nerve supply to the soft and hard
palates?

105 Describe the bed of the palatine tonsil and its
arterial supply.

106 Describe the ring of lymphoid tissue in the
upper pharynx (Waldeyer's ring).

107 Describe the fibres both passing through and
synapsing in the pterygopalatine ganglion.

108 Why are the constrictor muscles often likened
to a 'stack of flowerpots'?

109 The inferior constrictor has two parts. What is
the difference in their origins?

110   Does the pharyngeal plexus supply all the muscles of the pharynx, palate and tongue?

111   Describe the motor contribution of the glossopharyngeal nerve and the one and only muscle it supplies directly.

112   Which muscles are involved in elevation of the hyoid during swallowing?

113   What are the valleculae?

Applied questions

114   Why are anterior epistaxes common and why are posterior epistaxes often more difficult to stop and may even require arterial ligation?

115   Why should a patient complaining about toothache be asked about recent upper respiratory tract infections and have his frontal sinuses examined?

116   During a posterior rhinoscopy examination, which structures would you hope to see?

117   What differences are there between the auditory (Eustachian, pharyngotympanic) tube of a child and that of an adult and how does this help explain the frequency of middle ear disease in children?

118   To test which cranial nerves do you tickle the soft palate and make the patient 'gag'?

119   Why might a child with recurrent ear infections benefit from an adenoidectomy?

120   Your patient has tonsillitis. Which single palpable lymph node would you expect to be enlarged?

121   If you excise the epiglottis, what consequences do you think might develop?

122   To what does the term 'hypopharynx' refer and, as it is not an uncommon site of cancerous growth, how could you examine it?

123 A pharyngeal pouch may occur, particularly in the elderly. What is its anatomical explanation?

124 Where is the most likely site for a fish bone to impact in the pharynx?

G **Larynx**
   Thyroid
   Anterior triangle of the neck

Information questions

125 Describe the origins of the styloid process, stylomandibular ligament, hyoid bone and laryngeal cartilages.

126 Describe the laryngeal skeleton.

127 Describe the sphincter mechanisms of the larynx that protect the trachea from the entry of foreign bodies.

128 Which is the most vital muscle in the larynx?

129 Describe both the motor and the sensory nerve supply to the larynx.

130 Name the anatomical structure which is called the 'Adam's apple'.

131 What is the levator glandulae thyroideae?

132 Describe the blood supply of the thyroid gland.

133 Define the borders of the anterior triangle of the neck.

134 Where are the prevertebral and the deep cervical 'investing' fascia situated?

135 Describe the action of the infrahyoid and suprahyoid muscles on swallowing.

136 Why is the ansa cervicalis so called?

137 Name the branches of the external carotid artery and its two terminal arteries.

138 Why is the Adam's apple more prominent in the male, and what growth changes in the larynx accompany deepening of the male voice?

139 You are shown a lateral soft tissue x-ray of the neck and notice that some of the laryngeal skeleton appears as dense as bone and non-translucent. Can you suggest a reason for this occurrence?

140 At which vertebral levels do the following normally lie: hyoid, thyroid isthmus and cricoid cartilage?

141 When performing an indirect laryngoscopy, what do you think might be visible?

142 Discuss the effects on breathing and speech of an external laryngeal nerve palsy, and a bilateral paralysis of the recurrent laryngeal nerves.

143 In an anteroposterior tomogram x-ray of larynx, can you explain why the vocal cords are normally together?

144 What is the difference between tracheostomy and laryngotomy, and which important structures would you encounter performing these procedures?

145 Why does the inferior thyroid artery have such a tortuous course?

146 Why does the thyroid gland move on swallowing?

147 Why should a surgeon about to perform a thyroidectomy examine the vocal cords?

148 A patient sticks out his tongue and you notice that a swelling in the midline, above the hyoid, rises. What embryological abnormality do you suspect?

149 Why may a parathyroid gland be found within the thymus in a retrosternal position?

150 What are the contents and surface markings of the carotid sheath?

151 Discuss how you would easily distinguish the internal from the external carotid artery in the neck on a carotid arteriogram.

152 What important nerves might be damaged in an overenthusiastic carotid arteriogram puncture?

H Mouth
  Tongue
  Teeth
  Mandible
  Sublingual and submandibular salivary
    glands

Information questions

153 Describe the boundaries of the vestibule.

154 Which nerves are involved in general sensation (e.g. touch) from the tongue?

155 Describe the nerves involved in taste.

156 Describe the tongue muscles.

157 Describe the relationship of the tongue to the thyroid gland during development.

158 What is the chorda tympani, and what fibres does it carry?

159 What teeth would you expect to find in the mouth of a 4-month-old child, 20-month-old child and a 12-year-old schoolboy?

160 Which nerves and glands are in direct contact with the mandible?

161 Describe the positions of the two parts of the submandibular gland.

162 Describe the pathway of secretomotor parasympathetic impulses from the superior salivary nucleus to the submandibular gland.

163 What is the relationship between the lingual nerve and the submandibular duct?

Applied questions

164 Why might a young baby present with a small fleshy tumour in the midline at the back of the tongue? Describe its likely histology.

165 Why is genioglossus muscle of importance in maintaining an airway in the unconscious patient?

166 Why might a patient with a carcinoma of the tongue complain of severe earache?

167 Describe why cancer of the tongue in the posterior third has a very bad reputation and reduced prognosis compared to that of the anterior two-thirds.

168 How might a patient present if she had a right hypoglossal nerve palsy?

169 Following extraction of the right lower wisdom tooth, a patient complained of a numb tongue and a metallic taste in the mouth. How can you explain this situation?

170 Why might a tumour of the middle ear cause abnormal sensations of taste?

171 In a group of 22-year-old students, how many teeth would you suppose the majority to have?

172 Why might a simple jaw fracture result in a numb lower lip?

173 Following removal of the submandibular gland for a cancerous growth, why might the patient have a 'drooped' lower lip?

174 Where do you think a radiologist would insert his cannula to do a sialogram of the submandibular gland?

I Posterior triangle of the neck
Occipital region

Information questions

175 Describe the floor of the posterior triangle.

176 Describe the borders and roof of the posterior triangle.

177 Where do lymph nodes lie on the side of the neck?

178 What sensory nerves emerge from the cervical plexus?

179 Where is the normal C1 dermatome situated?

Applied questions

180 Why may surgery in the inferior portion of the posterior triangle be very dangerous? What important structures might you encounter?

181 Why might a patient, following surgery for an abscess on the side of the neck, be unable to brush her hair?

182 Why might a known leprosy patient present with numbness over the lobule of the ear and a cord-like swelling along the posterior border of the sternomastoid muscle?

183 Why is it relatively easy for infection in the occipital region to spread intracranially?

184 What important structure lies in the floor of the suboccipital triangle?

J Root of the neck
Sympathetic trunk
First rib

Information questions

185 What is the surface marking of the pleura in the root of the neck?

186 What are the branches of the subclavian artery in the neck?

187 Describe the course of the vertebral artery.

188 Can you explain the obvious difference between the origins of right and left recurrent laryngeal nerves from their respective vagi?

189 What is the course of the thoracic duct from the cisterna chyli to the brachiocephalic vein?

190 Describe the formation and connections of the cervical sympathetic ganglia.

191 Describe the relationships of scalenus anterior, the phrenic nerve, transverse cervical artery and thoracic duct to each other.

192 Describe the relative positions of the lower trunk of the brachial plexus, subclavian vein and artery to the first rib.

193 How would you distinguish the first rib from any other rib?

Applied questions

194 Why might a brachiocephalic venous catheterisation be inadvisable on the left side?

195 Why might a gunshot wound in the region above the clavicle cause weakness in abduction of the shoulder?

196 Why is it dangerous to point the needle posteriorly when performing central venous catheterisation into the internal jugular, subclavian or brachiocephalic veins?

197 What is the stellate ganglion, and why might a cervical sympathectomy cause facial and ophthalmic signs (Horner's syndrome)?

198 What is a cervical rib, and how might it present in a patient?

K   Ear

Information questions

199   Describe the sensory supply to the pinna and the tympanic membrane.

200   Describe how sound is transmitted from the external ear to the fenestra vestibuli.

201   What is the important posterior relation of the mastoid antrum?

202   Describe the main features of the medial wall of the middle ear.

203   Describe the course of the VIIth cranial nerve within the petrous temporal bone.

204   What are the three small branches from the VIIth cranial nerve given off in the petrous temporal bone, and what is their functional importance?

205   Describe the membranous labyrinth.

206   What is the relationship between the three semicircular canals?

207   Describe the cochlea.

Applied questions

208   Describe the external ear to the tympanic membrane and explain from where the wax comes.

209   What would you expect to see on the right tympanic membrane in a normal otoscopic examination?

210   How do you straighten the external auditory meatus in an adult or in an infant when trying to see the tympanic membrane?

211   When clearing their ears with a cotton-wool stick, why do some people start coughing and a few people even vomit?

212 Why should a Ramsay Hunt syndrome cause vesicles in the external auditory meatus?

213 A patient with abnormally sensitive hearing (hyperacusis), an unusual taste in the mouth, facial weakness, deafness and vertigo may well have a lesion in which region?

214 A young child presents in your clinic with a perforation of the ear drum and a large swelling in the mastoid region. Two days later he is brought into the clinic obviously very ill, drowsy and, from the mother's description, having just had convulsions. What do you fear has happened to his infection?

215 Can you explain why air hostesses give you sweets to eat at take off and landing?

UPPER LIMB

A Axilla
   Brachial plexus
   Breast

Information questions

216 What is the axillary sheath?

217 Describe the base, apex, walls and contents of the axilla.

218 Describe the branches from the posterior and medial cords of the brachial plexus.

219 Describe the formation of the cords of the brachial plexus.

220 What is the distribution of dermatomes C5 and C6?

221 Describe the muscle bed of the female breast and how the normal breast maintains its rounded contour.

222 Describe the lymphatic drainage of the breast.

223 An invasive melanoma of the finger might spread to which region of the axilla?

224 Why should a cervical rib cause loss of muscle bulk in the hand?

225 A small child was swung around very fast in a circle by his arms and afterwards was found to have sustained a traction injury to the upper trunk of the brachial plexus (Erb's palsy). In what position would the damaged arm be held and why?

226 A patient complained that, following a difficult radical mastectomy, her scapula stuck out like a wing when she pushed open a door. Can you explain why?

227 You find that a patient still has sensation on the upper aspect of the shoulder following a gunshot wound in the region of the brachial plexus. Why might this be possible?

228 Why is an intramuscular injection posteriorly into the deltoid muscle potentially very dangerous?

229 A patient presents in your clinic with wasting of all the intrinsic muscles of his right hand. He explains that he has suffered from this since the day he fell off his motor-cycle. You diagnose a Klumpke's palsy. What is the anatomical explanation?

230 What anatomical structure accounts for the fact that breast disease often causes dimpling and tethering of the skin?

231 An intradermal swelling and pitting (peau d'orange) is occasionally seen in cancers of the breast. What anatomical explanation can you suggest for this phenomenon?

232 What features might you expect to see on breast examination of a pregnant woman?

233   A patient has malignant change in the skin surrounding her nipple (Paget's disease). To which lymph nodes might metastases spread?

B   Scapular region
Shoulder joint and girdle

Information questions

234   Describe the axillary artery and the arterial anastomoses around the scapula.

235   How would you distinguish between a right and a left clavicle?

236   Discuss the muscles involved in abduction of the arm to 180°.

237   What is the most important function of the coracoclavicular ligament?

238   What is the relationship of muscles in the intertubercular (bicipital) groove?

239   What factors contribute to the stability of the shoulder joint? Why should it dislocate so relatively easily?

240   Describe the rotator cuff muscles and their importance.

Applied questions

241   What are the effects of a torn supraspinatus tendon?

242   What nerve might be damaged in a fracture of the neck of the humerus or a dislocation of the shoulder?

243   Where is the anatomical neck as distinct from the surgical neck of the humerus?

244   Why might a fractured clavicle appear with its medial third elevated and lateral two-thirds depressed and pulled anteriorly?

245 After a car accident your patient has a painful shoulder. Why might you ask especially for an axial x-ray of the shoulder in abduction?

C Upper arm
   Elbow joint
   Cubital fossa

Information questions

246 Describe the venous drainage of the upper limb.

247 Describe the courses and relationships, in the upper arm, of the median nerve and brachial artery. What happens to each as they leave the cubital fossa?

248 What nerves are related to the humerus itself?

249 Describe the course of the cephalic vein in the arm.

250 What is the carrying angle?

251 The elbow joint is really three different joints. What movements occur at each?

252 Describe the muscles involved in pronation and supination. Where is the axis of rotation?

253 Where can you normally palpate the ulnar and the superficial branch of the radial nerve?

254 Describe the boundaries, roof, floor and contents of the cubital fossa.

255 Discuss the origins and distribution of the anterior and posterior interosseous nerves.

256 Describe the course of the radial nerve.

Applied questions

257 Describe the landmarks you would use in finding the brachial artery either to measure blood pressure or to obtain arterial blood.

258 Why did a patient who had to use crutches for a
week complain of difficulty in gripping things
and a weakness at his wrists?

259 A famous boxer attempted an uppercut on an
opponent and missed. Afterwards he noticed
pain in the shoulder, a 'blacksmith's bulge' for
his biceps and difficulty in turning a door
handle. How do you explain this anatomically?

260 A supracondylar fracture of the humerus is a
common injury in children who fall out of trees.
Why might this be a serious injury and why
may it possibly cause severe loss of muscle
tissue distal to the fracture?

261 A farmer falls over and cuts his ulnar nerve at
the elbow. What functional effects will this have
and how will his hand look some months later?

262 A young boy is dragged by the arm from an
ice-cream shop and then complains of pain in
the forearm. There is a small hollow 1 cm distal
to the lateral epicondyle. What is your diagnosis and why does this happen more often in
children?

263 Why do screws have a right-hand thread?

264 Miners, and very occasionally nowadays
students, may present with a swelling over the
olecranon. What is it and how is it caused?

265 In a dislocated elbow joint, how would feeling
the epicondyles and olecranon help in differential diagnosis from a supracondylar fracture?

266 On flexing his elbow, a patient complains of
tingling in the little finger. An orthopaedic
surgeon cures the problem by doing what procedure to which nerve?

267 A student has performed a clumsy venepunc-
ture, pierced the 'grâce à Dieu' fascia and left
the patient with a large expanding mass in the
cubital fossa. Can you explain what has happened?

268 What is similar about palmaris longus and peroneus tertius?

23

D Forearm
Wrist joint

Information questions

269 What muscles attach at the common extensor origin?

270 Describe the wrist joint and its movements.

271 Abduction and adduction of the wrist are achieved by which muscles?

272 Why is it difficult to make a strong grip with a flexed wrist?

273 Describe the 'anatomical snuffbox'.

Applied questions

274 Which area of skin (dermatome) would be affected by a C6 herpes zoster infection?

275 What is the functional difference between injury to the ulnar nerve at the wrist and at the elbow?

276 An attempted suicide cuts his wrist fairly deeply. After repair of the arteries, which other important structures would you also wish to test and how would you do this?

277 A young woman falls on the outstretched hand and six weeks later complains of pain deep in the 'anatomical snuffbox' on palpation. Why should you x-ray her wrist?

278 You notice in 'cops and robbers' films that, to make a person drop a knife, the defender often hits the attacker's hand into acute flexion. Why is this a very sensible move?

E Hand

Information questions

279 Describe the arrangement of muscles and tendons attached to the middle finger.

280   Describe the flexor synovial sheaths.

281   What are the intrinsic muscles of the hand?

282   What are the dermatome and the myotome of T1?

283   Describe the nerve supply to the thenar and hypothenar muscles.

284   Describe the function of the interossei and lumbricals. Why do you need them to write properly?

285   How do the ulnar and the radial artery contribute to the blood supply of the hand? Give the surface markings of the palmar arches.

286   Describe which lymph node groups might become involved in an infection in the skin of the hand.

287   Describe the movements of the thumb. What is their relationship to those of the fingers?

Applied questions

288   An old woman falls downstairs and sustains a mid-shaft fracture of the humerus, damaging the radial nerve in the spiral groove. What are the effects, both motor and sensory, on the hand and wrist?

289   In the hand, which nerve lesion would be most serious, and why?

290   Why do the ring and little fingers have fixed flexion contractures in Dupuytren's disease?

291   In compression of the structures below the flexor retinaculum at the wrist (carpal tunnel syndrome), why is there weakness of the thenar muscles but normal sensation over the skin of the same region?

292   How might a swelling proximal to the wrist joint be connected with infection in the tip of the thumb (tenosynovitis)?

293 A patient with leprosy has a wasted hand with 'guttering', a positive Froment's sign, and a claw of his ring and little fingers. What lesion is responsible?

294 Where would you perform an operation for Raynaud's disease of the hands? What might be its effects?

THORAX

A Thoracic wall
  Intercostal spaces
  Ribs
  Sternum
  Joints of the thorax

Information questions

295 What is meant by the terms 'pump handle' and 'bucket handle' respiration?

296 Why is the vertebral level of T4 an important anatomical landmark?

297 When does one normally use the external inter-costal muscles?

298 Describe the arterial supply and venous drain-age of the left fifth intercostal space.

299 Describe the anatomy of an intercostal nerve.

300 What is meant by 'false' and 'floating' ribs?

301 Describe the articulations of the right sixth rib with the vertebral column.

Applied questions

302 At which vertebral levels would one normally find the jugular notch, manubriosternal joint and inferior angle of the scapula?

303 A young Australian surfer presents with a small malignant melanoma on his back just medial to the inferior tip of the scapula. Which lymph

nodes would you wish to examine or biopsy to detect any spread of the disease?

304 A paraumbilical tattoo, as practised by South American Indians, becomes infected. Which lymph nodes do you think will feel tender?

305 An anaesthetist performs a successful T5 nerve block. Why would there be no sensory loss on the anterior chest wall?

306 Why might a patient with tuberculosis of the T9 vetebral body present with abdominal pain?

307 A young man presents with shingles in a line just at the level of his umbilicus. Which branch of which spinal nerve is affected?

308 In coarctation of the aorta, the arterial blood finds a collateral circulation. Which vessels do you think are involved, and, after some time, what x-ray abnormalities might you see?

309 Following interchondral subluxation of the ninth costal cartilage, which muscles might go into spontaneous contraction?

310 Why does the first rib, on a chest x-ray, often look as if it ends in mid-air?

311 Why might a cervical rib cause pain in the region of the medial epicondyle of the humerus?

312 You are shown an x-ray of the sternum in which at least three separate sternebrae are visible. How old is the patient, approximately?

B Pleural cavity
Lungs

Information questions

313 Describe the surface marking of the dome of the pleura.

314 Compare and contrast the nerve supply of the parietal and visceral layers of the pleura.

315 What is the pulmonary ligament?

316 What is meant by the term 'pleural cavity'?

317 Describe the lymphatic drainage of the lungs.

 318 What are the costodiaphragmatic and costo-mediastinal recesses?

319 What is a bronchopulmonary segment?

320 Describe the position of the middle lobe of the right lung. To what does this lobe correspond on the left?

321 Describe the arterial supply and venous drainage of the main bronchi.

Applied questions

322 Why does pleurisy often mimic other causes of upper abdominal pain?

323 If the pleura is ruptured, what are the immediate consequences?

324 You are informed that a patient has a pleural effusion. Where is the fluid situated?

325 How would you drain the pleural cavity of air, and through which structures would your needle penetrate?

326 Why might it be useful to know the surface marking of the dome of the pleura prior to neck vein catheterisation?

327 Why might an unlucky central venous catheterisation cause a chylothorax?

328 Where on a bronchogram might you see the apicoposterior segmental bronchus?

329 You are told your patient has an apical basal pneumonia. Where on the chest would you expect to hear abnormal sounds with your stethoscope?

330 Your patient has unwanted bronchial **secretions** in her posterior basal segments. Into what position would she be best placed to aid postural drainage?

331 Why might a spreading apical carcinoma of the lung cause pain in the little finger and a partial drooping upper eyelid of the same side?

C Heart
Pericardium

Information questions

332 Describe the conduction mechanism of the heart.

333 Describe the venous drainage of the heart.

334 Why are the coronary arteries so called?

335 Describe the course and distribution of the left coronary artery.

336 What is the function of the papillary muscles and chordae tendineae?

337 What vessels drain into the right atrium?

338 How many layers does the pericardium possess?

339 Describe the nerve supply to the parietal pericardium.

340 Where would you find the transverse and oblique sinuses of the pericardium?

341 What important structures are embedded in the fibrous pericardium?

Applied questions

342 What are the surface markings of the heart valves, and why does one not listen at these sites to hear them best?

343 On a plain posteroanterior chest x-ray, what structures form the borders of the heart shadow?

344 Why is the pain of myocardial infarction not felt over the apex beat?

345 Why may one find an anatomically patent foramen ovale in a normal subject with no functional deficit?

346 During a knife fight your patient was stabbed medial to the apex beat in the fifth left intercostal space near to the sternum. Which chamber would you expect to have been lacerated?

347 Your patient has heart block. What x-ray might reveal an abnormality related to the normal functioning of the atrioventricular node?

348 What use would a lateral view barium swallow x-ray be to a physician investigating a patient with mitral valve disease?

349 Why has the right atrium both smooth and rough areas?

350 On x-ray, your patient has a globular-looking heart shadow due to a pericardial effusion. In draining the pericardium via the costoxiphoid approach, what structures would you encounter?

D Anterior mediastinum
   Posterior mediastinum
   Superior mediastinum

Information questions

351 Describe the limits and contents of the anterior mediastinum.

352 Describe the origin, course and termination of the thoracic duct.

353 What is the origin of the splanchnic nerves, and what fibres do they contain?

354 What is the relationship between structures running vertically and those running horizontally in the posterior mediastinum?

355 What is the blood supply of the oesophagus?

356 What are the grey and white rami communicantes?

357 What is the stellate ganglion?

358 What are the contents of the superior mediastinum?

359 What is the ligamentum arteriosum?

360 Describe the origin and course of the left and right recurrent laryngeal nerves.

Applied questions

361 Which glandular organ may appear as a swelling in the anterior mediastinum, and what symptoms do you think it may cause?

362 Why do the trachea and main bronchi not collapse during the negative pressure of inspiration?

363 Why might a patient with an apical carcinoma of the lung present with a hoarse voice?

364 Your patient has a carcinoma of the lower oesophagus. Where would you expect any metastases to spread?

365 What normal structures cause indentations of the anterior oesophageal wall as seen on a lateral barium swallow film?

366 Why should you be interested in the venous supply of the lower oesophagus when presented with an alcoholic young Frenchman who has vomited 2 litres of blood?

367 Why should tracheo-oesophageal abnormalities be not infrequent in the newborn child?

368 At an exciting movie, a young boy throws a peanut into the air and, attempting to catch it in his mouth, inhales it. Into which bronchus is it likely to pass?

ABDOMEN

A Anterior abdominal wall
   Inguinal canal
   Testes and scrotum

Information questions

369 Describe the nine surface regions of the abdomen and how they are derived.

370 Where are the linea alba, linea semilunaris and arcuate line?

371 What are the differences in the posterior rectus sheath above and below the umbilicus?

372 Why is L1 a classic anatomical landmark?

373 Which potentially weak regions of the anterior abdominal wall are sites for herniae?

374 Describe the layers of the superficial fascia of the abdomen and explain why there is no deep fascia.

375 How is the conjoint tendon related to the inguinal canal?

376 What is the tunica albuginea?

377 What single structure is easily palpable within the spermatic cord, and from where does it derive its blood supply?

378 Describe the course of a sperm from testis to urethra.

379 What is unusual about the superficial fascia of the scrotum?

380 What remnants of the paramesonephric ducts remain in the adult male?

381 Why should a person, after a paraumbilical tattoo, have swollen lymph nodes in both groins and both axillae?

382 What anatomical differences are there between an indirect and a direct inguinal hernia, and why do you think baby boys may present with indirect herniae?

383 Where is McBurney's point, and for which operation is it a landmark?

384 What is a gridiron incision? Describe the direction of fibres in each layer.

385 To drain off excess fluid within the peritoneal cavity (ascites), a trocar and cannula is used. Where would you insert it and through which structures would it pass?

386 Why should the rectus abdominis muscle be retracted laterally during a paramedian incision?

387 Describe the anatomical structures encountered during a Pfannenstiel incision.

388 A patient has a blocked inferior vena cava. How will blood return to the right atrium from the lower half of the body?

389 Why might your patient, following an inguinal hernia repair, complain of a pain in his scrotum?

390 Where does a kick in the testes hurt?

391 How and why does the lymphatic drainage of the scrotum and of the testes differ?

392 What are a hydrocele and a varicocele, and why is aspiration of a hydrocele often only of temporary relief?

393 To perform a vasectomy, which layers of the spermatic cord must one incise?

394 What structures does the gubernaculum become in the adult female?

B Peritoneal cavity

Information questions

395 In which of the nine zones of the abdomen are the following to be found: stomach, spleen, liver and ileocaeal valve or orifice?

396 Which of the following structures are normally intraperitoneal: pancreas, spleen, kidney, liver, transverse colon and duodenum?

397 What is the difference between A mesentery and THE mesentery?

398 The epiploic foramen (Winslow) leads from the greater sac into what structure?

399 What are the walls of the omental bursa?

400 What is the falciform ligament and what structure lies within its free border?

401 How many layers of peritoneum are involved in the formation of the greater omentum?

402 Describe the position and form of the lesser omentum. What lies within its free border?

403 Where are the triangular and coronary ligaments?

404 What lies within the lienorenal ligament?

405 Who normally have openings into their peritoneal cavity?

406 What embryological structures do the median and medial umbilical ligaments represent?

Applied questions

407 What structures form within the ventral mesentery of the foregut?

408 What is ascites and, anatomically, where does it lie?

409 If your finger were in the lesser sac (omental bursa), what structures would be posterior to it?

410 Why is the epiploic foramen (Winslow) very useful to the surgeon during a bloody cholecystectomy operation?

411 Why is a twisting of the bowel (volvulus) relatively common in the sigmoid colon but very rare in the descending colon?

412 Why is the pain of early appendicitis generalised and paraumbilical in site, whereas later on in the course of the disease it is localised to the right iliac fossa?

413 What are the subphrenic spaces, and why are they important?

C Gastrointestinal tract
Stomach
Small and large intestine

Information questions

414 Where do the vagi lie on entering the abdominal cavity?

415 Describe the innervation of the stomach.

416 Describe the structures lying in the 'stomach bed'.

417 Which major artery and its branches supply the foregut?

418 Describe the lymphatic drainage of the stomach.

419 How would you distinguish between jejunum and ileum?

420 How does the small intestine receive its autonomic nerve supply?

421 What are the distinguishing features of the large intestine compared to the small intestine?

422 Describe the arterial blood supply to the transverse colon.

423 Where is the origin of the sigmoid mesocolon?

Applied questions

424 What is congenital pyloric stenosis and when does it usually present?

425 A surgeon wishes to cut both vagus nerves (vagotomy). Where do you think they are most easily found in the abdomen?

426 Why might a patient with a cancer of the stomach present with obstructed pancreatic drainage?

427 What is the 'policeman of the abdomen'?

428 Under what circumstances might air appear in the peritoneal cavity, and how might this be seen radiologically?

429 A diverticulum (Meckel) is occasionally found on the antimesenteric border of the ileum. What is it?

430 Why might a remnant of the vitellointestinal duct present problems for a surgeon?

431 What radiological features distinguish large from small bowel?

432 Why is the caecum sometimes found in the right hypochondrium?

433 Which region of the large bowel is most likely to suffer from ischaemia and why?

434 Diverticulosis of the colon is a common disease. Is there an anatomical explanation for the sites of development of this problem?

D Pancreas
   Spleen
   Duodenum

Information questions

435 Why does the superior mesenteric artery appear to pierce the pancreas?

436 What is the relationship between the tail of the pancreas and the spleen?

437 Describe the four parts of the duodenum and their relation to the vertebral column and the head of the pancreas.

438 Describe the venous drainage of the spleen.

439 What do the splenic notches tell you about the spleen's development?

440 Describe the shape and surface markings of the spleen.

441 Describe the splenic artery.

Applied questions

442 Can you explain, from your knowledge of embryology, why there is commonly a main pancreatic duct (Wirsung) which opens with the common bile duct as well as a subsidiary duct (Santorini) which opens into the duodenum superiorly?

443 How may either the biliary or the pancreatic ducts be viewed radiologically?

444 Why should a cancer of the head of the pancreas cause a patient to be jaundiced?

445 Why might a posterior pancreatic tumour cause venous obstruction of the lower limbs?

446 A patient involved in a car accident ruptures his spleen, and whilst recumbent complains of left shoulder tip pain. How do you explain this symptom anatomically?

447 Why is the duodenum relatively difficult to mobilise during surgery?

E Liver
   Biliary system
   Portal venous system

Information questions

448 Name the lobes of the liver. Are they functionally distinct?

449 Describe the blood supply of the liver.

450 What is the 'bare area' of the liver? Describe its boundaries.

451 Can you expect to feel the liver in a normal person?

452 Describe, in the fetus, the path taken by blood from the umbilicus to the inferior vena cava, and how this changes after birth.

453 What structures lie in the porta hepatis?

454 Describe the extrahepatic biliary tree.

455 Describe the most common arrangement in the formation of the portal vein.

456 Where are the main sites of portosystemic venous anastomoses?

Applied questions

457 In performing a liver biopsy, why should a pneumothorax be a not uncommon complication?

458 Why must the patient hold his breath during a liver biopsy?

459 What is a Riedel's lobe and why is it worth knowing about?

460 By what technique could you view the venous drainage of the liver?

461 How can you explain obstruction of the bowel due to gallstones?

462 Inflammation of the gall bladder may present as pain felt in which region?

463 Why might a patient with a long history of gallstones suddenly become jaundiced?

F Kidney
   Ureter
   Suprarenal gland

Information questions

464 Describe the anterior and posterior relations of the kidneys.

465 Describe the 'capsules' of the kidney.

466 A pelvic kidney may derive its blood supply from which artery?

467 What major difference is there between the tributaries of the right and left renal veins?

468 Describe the normal flow of urine from a lesser calyx to the bladder.

469 What is the blood supply to the ureters?

470 Describe the relationship of structures at the hilum of the kidney.

471 Describe the relations of the suprarenal glands.

472 What is the connection between the suprarenal cortex and the sympathetic nervous system?

Applied questions

473 How could you explain the occurrence of a left-sided varicocele in a man with a palpable abdominal mass and blood in his urine (haematuria)?

474 Describe the structures encountered in performing a lower pole renal biopsy.

475 What are the surface markings of the kidneys, and what explains their difference in position?

476 Why might a patient have a pneumothorax after a renal biopsy?

477 Why should a horseshoe kidney be situated at a lower level than the normal organ?

478 How might the upper urinary tract be viewed radiologically?

479 What are the classic markings of the right ureter on an abdominal x-ray?

480 Which relatively narrow sites of the ureter would you check for the impaction of stones?

G Posterior abdominal wall
     Diaphragm

Information questions

481 Which nerves exit the psoas muscle along its lateral border?

482 Name the paired arterial branches of the abdominal aorta.

483 What are the tributaries of the inferior vena cava, and what makes them asymmetrical?

484 What is the hypogastric plexus?

485 Describe the lymph nodes of the posterior abdominal wall.

486 What is the relationship of the common iliac artery, ureter and testicular vessels at the brim of the pelvis?

487 Explain the relationships to each other of the following structures: ureter, testicular vessels, psoas muscle and right colic artery.

488 What are the origins of the diaphragm?

489 What are the median, medial and lateral arcuate ligaments?

490 From which main structures is the diaphragm formed and how does this explain its motor and sensory nerve supply?

491 Which structures pass through the diaphragm and at what approximate vertebral levels?

Applied questions

492 What is the solar plexus, and if you receive a blow to this region what happens?

493 A young Indian boy complains of a swelling in his lumbar spine and, more recently, a swelling in the groin. Anatomically, how can you connect these two symptoms?

494 On which x-ray would you hope to find a cisterna chyli, and what is its function?

495 Describe the surface markings of the abdominal aorta.

496 In a patient with a testicular tumour, where would you wish to examine lymph nodes for suspected metastases?

497 Discuss the likely sites of both congenital and acquired herniae of the diaphragm.

498 Where do you think pain is felt after an injury to the central portion of the diaphragm?

499 Through which part of the diaphragm does the inferior vena cava pass, and why must this be so?

PELVIS AND PERINEUM

A Bones and ligaments
   Sexual differences

Information questions

500 What are the true and the false pelvis?

501 Given a bony pelvis, how would you position it correctly?

502 What are the pelvic inlet (brim) and the pelvic outlet?

503 What type of joints are the pubic symphysis and sacroiliac joints?

504 What is the relationship between the lacunar and inguinal ligaments?

505 How might the greater sciatic notch help you distinguish a male from a female pelvis?

506 What creates the difference between the male and the female bony pelvis?

Applied questions

507 What bony landmarks do you think are used when performing a pudendal nerve block during labour?

508 What are the true and diagonal conjugates?

509 Why might the sacral hiatus prove a very useful landmark for the anaesthetist?

510 The 'dimples of Venus' are easily seen when watching young women in bikinis! What are they, and for what anatomical landmarks are they a useful guide?

511 On vaginal examination, you find a woman to have a subpubic angle of about 60°. What does this tell you about her pelvis?

512 On vaginal examination in early pregnancy, you estimate your patient's ischial spines to be 8 cm apart. As her obstetrician, about what might you worry?

513 What are the normal measurements of the pelvic brim in a woman?

B Perineum
Male and female urogenital regions

Information questions

514 With what is Colles' fascia of the perineum continuous over the anterior abdominal wall?

515 Describe the main branches of the pudendal nerve.

516 Describe the three divisions of the male urethra and the two which are within the perineum.

517 What structures lie within the deep perineal pouch or space?

518 What muscles lie within the superficial perineal space or pouch?

519 Though artificial, what are the boundaries of the urogenital triangle?

520 Why is the dorsum of the penis so described?

521 What is the perineal body or central tendon of the perineum, and to which structures is it attached?

522 Where would you find the bulbourethral glands (Cowper) and what is their female homologue?

523 Describe the areas of drainage to the superficial inguinal lymph nodes.

Applied questions

524 How would you identify the site of the perineal membrane on a male urethrogram?

525 On a pelvic examination, where would you find an inflamed greater vestibular gland (Bartholin)?

526 Which are the widest and narrowest parts of the male urethra?

527 After rectal surgery, why are some men unable to ejaculate?

528 What do you think might be the consequences of a ruptured perineal body?

529 If the urethra in the superficial perineal space is ruptured, to where does the urine go?

530 What is hypospadias, and how does its occurrence help explain the development of the penile urethra in the male?

43

531 While performing a cystoscopy on a male patient, where is the most likely site for the tip of the instrument to wedge?

532 What is circumcision, and why should special care be taken when performing surgery around the frenulum?

C Pelvic floor
   Rectum
   Anal triangle

Information questions

533 Describe the levator ani.

534 Why is the ischiorectal fossa poorly named?

535 What are the internal and external anal sphincters and how are they innervated?

536 Describe the blood supply of the rectum and anus.

537 What are the rectal valves or transverse folds?

Applied questions

538 What have the pectinate line and hymen in common?

539 The pectinate line demarcates the proctodeum and cloaca of the embryo. How is this relevant to understanding metastases from an anal carcinoma?

540 What is the embryological explanation of an imperforate anus?

541 In performing a rectal examination on a male or female, what structures might you normally feel?

542 Why may haemorrhoids be associated with cirrhosis of the liver, and, if injected in the correct region, cause no pain?

543 What is the lithotomy position? Describe the boundaries of the anal triangle in this position.

544 What is the major content of the ischiorectal fossa, and why is it often a site of abscess formation?

D Male pelvic organs

Information questions

545 Into where do the ejaculatory ducts open?

546 How is the bladder innervated?

547 Describe the branches of the internal iliac artery.

548 The prostate has how many capsules?

549 Describe the peritoneal coverings of the rectum.

550 Describe the boundaries of the trigone. What type of receptors are particularly numerous in this region?

551 What is the verumontanum?

Applied questions

552 What remnants of the paramesonephric ducts are there in the adult male?

553 What is the clinical significance of drainage from the prostatic venous plexus?

554 Why should an enlarged prostate gland cause retention of urine?

555 What structures are normally visible on a vaso-gram x-ray?

556 A man complains of passing blood in his urine (haematuria) and, at the end of micturition, a very severe pain at the tip of the penis. With regard to the anatomy of the bladder, what comments can you make?

557 Why do you not develop peritonitis after a suprapubic catheterisation of a really full bladder?

558 In which normal people might one expect to percuss or palpate a bladder?

E Female pelvic organs

Information questions

559 From where does the ovary receive its blood and nerve supply?

560 What is the homologue of the round ligament of the uterus in the male embryo?

561 What is a retroflexed, retroverted uterus?

562 Describe the uterine tubes and their relationship to the broad ligament.

563 Describe the lymphatic drainage from the uterus.

564 What are the urachus and the obliterated umbilical artery called in the adult?

565 Describe the contents of the broad ligament.

566 What are the fornices of the vagina?

567 Describe the peritoneum of the female pelvis in contrast to that of the male.

568 What supports the uterus?

Applied questions

569 During what examination might one, by chance, feel pathology of the ureters?

570 What structures can one normally palpate during a bimanual pelvic examination?

571 During a hysterosalpingogram, contrast medium is seen to flow into the rectouterine pouch

(Douglas). What does this tell you about this woman's anatomy?

572 Name three structures—all remnants of the mesonephric ducts—which may, in the adult female, give rise to cystic swellings.

573 Why may an amateur abortionist accidentally kill his or her patients, due to peritonitis?

574 Why do some women experience paraumbilical pain about 14 days prior to menstruation?

575 Can you explain an abdominal pregnancy?

576 What consequences might follow stretching of the cardinal and uterosacral ligaments?

577 To which lymph nodes would an ovarian tumour most likely metastasise?

LOWER LIMB

A Gluteal region
  Hip joint

Information questions

578 What converts the greater and lesser sciatic notches into foramina?

579 Describe the structures which exit from the greater sciatic foramen below the piriformis muscle.

580 What structures enter the lesser sciatic foramen from the greater sciatic foramen?

581 Describe the course of the sciatic nerve as far as its bifurcation into common peroneal and tibial branches.

582 Describe the ligaments of the hip joint. Why is hip extension limited to only about 15°?

583 Describe the muscles involved in abduction of the hip. What is their most important function in everyday life?

584 Which are the six small lateral rotator muscles of the hip?

Applied questions

585 When performing intramuscular injections into the gluteal region, what anatomical landmarks would you use to make sure you did not damage the sciatic nerve?

586 A patient with prolapsed intervertebral discs at L4/5 and L5/S1 complains of sciatica. Where will the pain be worst, and which dermatomes will you examine to test for loss of sensation?

587 Why does a patient with congenital dislocation of the hip have a 'dipping gait' (Trendelenburg) on walking?

588 Why should a subcapital fracture in the elderly often lead to avascular necrosis of the femoral head whilst a pertrochanteric fracture usually heals well with a pin and plate procedure?

589 Why, on examination of a patient with a fractured neck of femur, would you often find shortening of the limb and lateral rotation of the foot?

590 Why does it seem that a ballet dancer can extend the hip to 90°? What, in fact, is she doing?

B Femoral triangle
   Adductor compartment of thigh

Information questions

591 Describe the boundaries, roof, floor and contents of the femoral triangle.

592 Describe the quadriceps, their actions and why the vastus medialis has horizontal fibres to the patella.

593 Describe the adductor muscles and their innervation.

594 Describe the adductor (Hunter's, subsartorial) canal and its contents.

Applied questions

595 On examination, you find your patient has a small femoral hernia which is reducible. After reduction, which is often not possible in this type of hernia, your finger lies in the femoral canal. What structures lie deep, superficial, medial and lateral to your examining finger?

596 Where and how would you find the femoral vein to obtain venous blood in a collapsed patient?

597 Your patient has a saphena varix—where would you expect to find this swelling?

598 By observation alone, how could you tell the difference between a femoral and an indirect inguinal hernia?

599 The long saphenous vein is homologous to which vein of the arm?

600 A patient with an ulcer on the glans penis should have which lymph node group examined?

601 Why should a patient with a tumour within the psoas muscle complain of tingling in his big toe and numbness of the side of his buttock and thigh?

602 Why might a patient complain of pain and paraesthesiae in the medial side of the lower leg following stripping of the long saphenous vein for varicosities?

603 A butcher's knife slips and plunges into his thigh at the apex of the femoral triangle. Why is this likely to be particularly bloody?

C   Knee joint
   Popliteal fossa

Information questions

604 Describe the bursae around the knee joint. Which are in direct communication with the joint?

605 What is the function of the cruciate ligaments, and what happens to them in flexion and hyperextension?

606 Describe the menisci and their function.

607 Which hamstrings have an action on the knee joint?

608 Describe the muscles and nerves involved in the knee jerk.

609 Describe the boundaries, floor, roof and contents of the popliteal fossa.

610 Describe the functional importance of the popliteus muscle.

Applied questions

611 An 8-year-old boy comes into your surgery with a pain in his knee. Why would you examine thoroughly both his knee and his hip?

612 Footballers often have to undergo operations for removal of one or both menisci. Which one is the most common meniscus to be torn and why?

613 Why can a physician obtain a 'patella tap' on a knee joint containing an effusion?

614 What are 'housemaid's knee' and 'clergyman's knee'?

615 Why should women suffer from dislocation of the patella more commonly than men? Name three factors which normally prevent lateral dislocation.

616 Describe the development of the patella. How might this explain the appearance of what looks like a fracture in a normal person?

617 A partly decomposed skeleton of a baby is found. Why might an x-ray of the knee be an important piece of evidence in distinguishing whether the child had been stillborn or had died after a short extrauterine life?

618 Why might a 'locked' knee be the presenting sign of a torn meniscus?

619 Why is a popliteal pulse difficult to feel even in the normal individual?

620 What structures do you think may be the cause of a swelling in the region of the popliteal fossa?

621 Which tendons are easily palpable at the back of the knee?

622 A young man is crossing the road and is knocked down by a bus. On arriving at the hospital it is noticed that he has a very swollen lateral side of the knee and lower leg and that he cannot dorsiflex his foot. Can you explain his 'foot-drop'?

D Compartments of lower leg
Ankle joint

Information questions

623 Which muscles are found in the flexor and the extensor compartment of the leg? Which muscles have a separate, third, compartment?

624 Describe the muscles involved in plantar flexion and in dorsiflexion.

625 Describe the superficial venous drainage of the lower limbs.

626 Describe the tendons in the extensor compartment at the ankle joint.

627 What are the nerve supply and particular action of the peronei muscles?

628 Describe the retinacula. What is their function?

629 Describe the major ligaments of the ankle joint.

630 Describe the muscles and nerves involved in the ankle jerk.

631 How would you test separately the functions of soleus from gastrocnemius?

632 Why might stripping the short saphenous vein for varicose veins leave the patient with a tingling in his little toe?

633 How would you display radiologically the veins of the leg? Why might this be useful clinically?

634 You are called to an emergency where a patient requires an instant intravenous line. All his veins are collapsed so you take a scalpel and 'cut-down' on the long saphenous vein. Where would you hope to find it?

635 Whom do you think sustains a rupture of the tendo calcaneus most often? What do you think are the consequences?

636 Does everyone have both the dorsalis pedis and posterior tibial pulses present?

637 Why are ankles sprained more commonly whilst walking downstairs rather than when going upstairs?

638 In a sprained ankle that has a forced eversion injury, the deltoid ligament may tear. Why is this quite a serious situation?

639 What is a Pott's fracture of the ankle, and why do you think a third degree type may often require internal fixation?

E Foot
Posture and walking

Information questions

640 Give examples in the leg of a 'red' and a 'white' muscle. What functional significance have these terms?

641 Describe the four named peripheral nerves which supply sensation to the dorsum of the foot.

642 What muscles produce inversion and eversion, and at which joints do these movements take place?

643 Name the factors which maintain the arches of the foot.

644 Where is the line of gravity?

645 Describe the major muscle groups involved in normal walking, and their sequence of contractions.

646 An infected cut on the heel will cause tenderness in which lymph nodes?

Applied questions

647 In a severe sprain of the ankle, why is it not uncommon to find that the patient has an avulsion of the fifth metatarsal tuberosity?

648 What is talipes equinovarus, and in whom may it be commonly seen?

649 In flat foot (pes planus), which arch is particularly depressed?

650 Why should a patient, following poliomyelitis of the lower leg, present with a claw-foot (pes cavus)?

651 Why might a lumbar sympathectomy help a patient with occlusive arterial disease of the lower limb?

BACK

A Vertebral column
Joints and ligaments

Information questions

652 Discuss the characteristic features of typical cervical, thoracic and lumbar vertebrae.

653 Which cervical spinous process is the most easily palpated?

654 Where is the body of the atlas?

655 At what level do the iliac crests usually lie?

656 Why is movement in the lumbar region mainly flexion and extension?

657 What type of joint lies between vertebral bodies?

658 Describe the specialised ligaments of the atlantoaxial joint.

659 Which animals have a very strong ligamentum nuchae, and from what is it formed?

660 Describe the main ligaments attached to the body and spine of a thoracic vertebra.

661 Describe the position of the ligamenta flava. Why are they thus called?

Applied questions

662 What are kyphosis, scoliosis and lordosis?

663 What is spina bifida?

664 Why do you think the posterior superior iliac spines are a useful landmark for a doctor wishing to examine the bone marrow?

665 On an oblique view x-ray of the lumbar vertebrae, what is the 'scottie dog'?

666 Why should the cervical vertebrae be prone to dislocation in whiplash injuries?

667 What might be an immediate consequence of a fracture dislocation of the dens?

668 Why would injection of contrast medium into the vertebral artery above C6 prove extremely difficult?

669 Why might a sudden posterior prolapse of the nucleus pulposus between C2 and C3 prove fatal?

670 What structures are pierced on performing a cisternal puncture (cerebellomedullary cisterna)?

671 Which is the most frequent site of herniation of the nucleus pulposus, and what may be the consequences?

B Soft tissues of the back
Suboccipital region

Information questions

672 What are the main muscle groups forming the erector spinae?

673 Of which muscles is the transversospinalis group composed?

674 What is the nerve supply to all the deep back muscles?

675 What is unusual about the dorsal ramus of C1 (suboccipital nerve)?

676 Describe the contribution made by the ventral rami to the sensory supply of the back of the neck.

677 Describe the small muscles involved in atlanto-occipital and atlantoaxial movements.

678 What is the most vital structure in the suboccipital triangle?

679 What forms the roof and floor of the suboccipital triangle?

Applied questions

680 Where are the triangle of auscultation and the lumbar triangle?

681 Why is the vertebral venous plexus (Batson) of great importance in understanding the spread of prostatic malignancy?

682 Why might a left-sided leg pain (sciatica) and a low back ache be associated with spasm of the left lower erector spinae?

683 If a patient complained of pain on the outer side of the upper arm, which increased in intensity during neck movement, which cervical vertebrae would you wish to x-ray?

684 On a cervical spine x-ray, what might you look for in the soft tissue region of a patient with tingling in both forearms whilst carrying suitcases?

C Spinal meninges
   Epidural space

Information questions

685 Describe the denticulate ligaments.

686 What is the filum terminale and where does it terminate?

687 Where do the spinal cord and spinal theca normally terminate in an adult?

688 How many pairs of nerves are derived from the spinal cord?

689 What lies within the subarachnoid space?

690 What are the contents of the epidural (extra-dural) space in the normal adult?

691 How far laterally does the dural sheath extend?

Applied questions

692 On a myelogram, why does one often see contrast medium around the nerve roots?

693 Why is a lumbar puncture at the level of L2 potentially hazardous in an infant?

694 Why does the normal lateral erect myelogram have indentations on its anterior thecal margin, and for what reason are these checked?

695 The intervertebral foramen has bony and cartilaginous walls. Why is this of significance?

696 What structures would be encountered in performing a lumbar puncture just below the spine of L4?

3

Answers

HEAD AND NECK

A Information answers

1 The bones of the vault of the skull, being flat, are ossified in membrane. Those of the base of the skull are, in general, ossified in cartilage. Thus the frontal bone, parietal bone, the squamous parts of the occipital and temporal bones and the greater wings of the sphenoid are ossified in membrane, as are the facial bones, viz. maxilla, zygomatic, palatine, lacrimal bones and the vomer.
[A:207; B:551; H:19]

2 The temporal bone is in four parts at birth: the squamous, petrous, styloid process and tympanic parts. The petrous and styloid are developed in cartilage, the other two in membrane.
[A:295; B:563; H:28]

3 The frontal bone ossifies in membrane from two centres, one on each side. These two are separated at birth by a suture—the metopic suture—situated in the median sagittal plane.
[A:299; G:78; H:25]

4 The vertex is the highest point of the skull in the anatomical position. It is situated in the median sagittal plane between the two parietal bones. The inion is synonymous with the external occipital protuberance. This is a bony protuberance of the occipital bone in the midline, for the attachment of the ligamentum nuchae. Above each orbit is the supraciliary ridge which is more prominent in males. The two supraciliary ridges are joined across the midline by an elevation—the glabella. The crista galli is situated on the interior of the skull. It is a sharp upward projection of the ethmoid bone in the midline of the anterior cranial fossa. It separates

the cribriform plates and gives attachment to the falx cerebri.
[A:257, 274; G:79; H:17]

5 Immediately medial to the spine of the sphenoid is situated the junction between the bony and cartilaginous portions of the auditory tube (Eustachian, pharyngotympanic), which the spine therefore protects. Anteromedially is situated the foramen spinosum, for the middle meningeal artery, which is therefore also protected to a degree. A further important relationship is the opening of the carotid canal posteromedially.
[A:268, 288; F:541]

6 The sphenoid usually has six apertures through it. The optic canal lies between two roots of bone which join the body to the lesser wing. It connects the cranial cavity with the orbit and transmits the optic nerve and ophthalmic artery. Four further foramina lie in a semicircle on the medial aspect of the middle cranial fossa. Most anteriorly is the superior orbital fissure, connecting the fossa to the orbit and conducting the branches of the ophthalmic division of V, the trochlea abducens and oculomotor nerves, and superior ophthalmic vein. Behind the superior orbital fissure is the foramen rotundum. It conducts the maxillary division of V on its way to the pterygo-palatine fossa. Next is the foramen ovale, which transmits the mandibular division of V (both sensory and motor parts) and the lesser petrosal nerve. Most posterior is the foramen spinosum through which the middle meningeal vessels enter the skull. The pterygoid canal links the pterygopalatine fossa with the foramen lacerum. It is situated at the base of the pterygoid process. It conducts the nerve of the pterygoid canal containing both sympathetic and parasympathetic elements on their way to the sphenopalatine ganglion.
[A:288; F:606; G:733; H:30]

7 The diploic veins drain the diploic space. This is the marrow-containing portion of cancellous bone situated between the inner and outer layers of compact bone, in the bones of the vault of the skull. The diploic veins emerge to the exterior of the skull. There are usually four on each side: one frontal, two parietal and one occipital.
[A:691; G:720]

8 The emissary veins connect the intracranial venous sinuses with veins on the outside of the skull. They are <u>valveless</u> and therefore blood may flow in either direction in them. They are clinically important because they may transmit extracranial infection to the inside of the skull.
[A:698; C:863]

9 The conchae are projections of the lateral wall of the nose into the nasal cavity. They consist of a bony skeleton covered in mucous membrane. There are three conchae on either side, named superior, middle and inferior. The <u>superior</u> and <u>middle conchae are derived from</u> the <u>ethmoid bone</u>; the <u>inferior is a separate bone in its own right</u>.
[A:279, 301; F:579; G:7114]

10 The foramen lacerum is situated in the middle cranial fossa between the irregular apex of the petrous temporal bone and the sphenoid. As its name suggests, it is irregular in shape. In life it is filled with cartilage and fibrous tissue. Only a few small veins actually pass through it but the internal carotid artery passes directly over it during its tortuous passage into the skull.
[A:276, 271; C:794]

11 The word 'antrum' is frequently used to describe the maxillary air sinus. This is a pyramidal air-filled space located in the body of the maxilla and lined with respiratory epithelium. It communicates with the middle meatus of the nasal cavity via the hiatus semilunaris.
[A:305, 1095; C:924]

12 The joint between the basi-occiput and the basi-sphenoid is a cartilaginous joint of the synchondrosis variety. The two bones' growing edges are separated by a block of cartilage into which they both grow and eventually fuse. This joint resembles, therefore, the joints between long bones and their epiphyses. The cartilage of the basi-occiput/basi-sphenoid joint is obliterated and bony union occurs around the <u>twenty-fifth year</u>.
[A:286, 388; F:605]

A Applied answers

13 The most obvious differences are the open sutures and fontanelles which allow moulding

of the skull during delivery. The anterior fontanelle (bregma) is diamond-shaped and bounded by the developing frontal and parietal bones. The two frontal bones normally fuse, but occasionally persist in the adult as a metopic suture. The posterior fontanelle (lambda) is triangular-shaped and lies between the occipital and parietal bones. These two fontanelles close by 2 years and 9 months, respectively.

The general bony proportions are different, the facial skeleton being relatively tiny at birth and only enlarging during the first few years. The alveolar processes and paranasal air sinuses are only rudimentary at birth and expand during growth as do the mastoid air cells. These differential growth rates contribute to internal changes such as the shape and position of the auditory tube as well as the more obvious changes such as the rounded baby face becoming an elongated adult face. Less obvious differences include the structure of the external auditory meatus. In the newborn its walls are cartilaginous as far as the tympanic membrane whereas in the adult the medial part of the meatus is part of the temporal bone and is therefore bony.
[B:578; G:105, 1010; H:19]

14 The mastoid air cells do not develop until the second or third year, and consequently the relatively small size of the newborn mastoid leaves the facial nerve exposed as it exits the skull through the stylomastoid foramen. A superficially placed nerve is therefore easily damaged, especially during forceps delivery.
[H:20, 35; I:251]

15 The normal beard overlies the zygomatic portion of the temporal bone, zygomatic bone, the ramus, angle and body of the mandible and the maxilla. An extremely long beard may of course overlie the manubrium and sternum!
[G:77; H:11]

16 The pterion is the meeting point of temporal, parietal and frontal bones with the greater wing of the sphenoid bone. In the fetal skull it may be seen as a fontanelle, whereas in the adult it lies some 4 cm above the midpoint of the zygomatic arch. Immediately deep to this point lies the

middle meningeal artery and, more specifically, its anterior division, which may be lacerated in a direct blow causing a fracture injury to the side of the head. The bone is relatively thin in this area and an extradural haematoma may follow a direct hit with a missile such as a golf or cricket ball.
[B:561; G:723; H:11, 22]

17 They are hollow bones containing air-filled spaces. The mastoid air cells lead into the middle ear whilst the ethmoid, sphenoid and maxillary paranasal air sinuses all open into the lateral wall of the nasal cavity. These air spaces are thought to lighten the weight of the skull.
[H:21]

18 The hyoid bone is a U-shaped structure with a body and four horns (cornua). It is the uppermost platform of the laryngeal cartilages and is derived from second and third arch cartilages. It is suspended from the styloid process by stylohyoid ligaments and has attached to it some dozen or so small muscles. These connect the hyoid bone to the tongue, jaw, sternum, larynx and pharynx. Consequently, following hyoid trauma the fine balance of these muscles would be disturbed, causing problems in breathing, speaking and swallowing.
[B:579; G:786; H:33]

19 A fracture of the mandible may easily involve the inferior alveolar (dental) nerve which lies within the bone. Its terminal branches exit the bone through the mental foramen where they supply the mucous membrane of the lower lip and chin. (Remember what happens to your lip following an inferior alveolar nerve block whilst undergoing dental procedures!)
[G:781; H:38]

B Information answers

20 The anterior cranial fossa is situated anterior to the lesser wings of the sphenoid bone. The middle cranial fossa lies between the lesser wing of the sphenoid anteriorly and the two petrous temporal bones posteriorly. The frontal lobes of the brain occupy the anterior cranial

fossa, the temporal lobes the middle cranial fossa.
[A:273; B:570; H:17]

21 The clinoid processes form the margins of the sella turcica. They provide attachments for the tentorium cerebelli—the attached border being attached to the posterior clinoid processes, the free border being attached to the anterior processes. Between the processes is stretched the diaphragma sellae, the dural roof of the sella turcica. Within the sella lies the pituitary gland.
[A:274, 987; E:699; H:17]

22 The clivus is the inclined surface between the anterior part of the foramen magnum and the sella turcica. It is composed of the occipital bone posteroinferiorly and the sphenoid anterosuperiorly, with the synchondrosis between them. The medulla lies against the lower aspect of the clivus, the pons against the upper part.
[A:274, 286; F:487; H:17]

23 The jugular foramen lies in the posterior cranial fossa between the lower border of the petrous temporal bone and the occipital bone. It transmits the sigmoid sinus, which becomes the internal jugular vein on passing through the foramen. The inferior petrosal sinus descends in a groove between the petrous temporal and occipital bones, to enter the foramen. It passes through the foramen anterior to the sigmoid sinus, to enter the internal jugular vein. The IXth, Xth and XIth cranial nerves also leave the skull through the jugular foramen. The IXth nerve grooves the inferior border of the petrous temporal bone as it does so. These three nerves exit anterior to the sigmoid sinus. From anterior to posterior, they are arranged IX, X, XI.
[A:272; B:567; C:804]

24 In the neck, the hypoglossal nerve descends in the carotid sheath anterior to the vagus. At the lower border of the posterior belly of diagastric, it loops around the occipital artery and, turning anteriorly, crosses superficial to both carotid arteries. As it progresses, it crosses the loop of the lingual artery superficially, and comes to lie on the superficial aspect of the hyoglossus

64

muscle. It is unique in having this superficial relationship to the carotid arteries.
[A:1025; E:632; F:786]

25 In certain areas the arachnoid projects into the intracranial venous sinuses to form arachnoid granulations. These granulations serve to drain cerebrospinal fluid into the venous blood. They are particularly numerous around the superior sagittal sinus where they groove the skull, forming pits in the internal aspect. The superior sagittal sinus has lateral extensions in various places. These are termed lacunae. They, too, contain arachnoid granulations.
[A:692, 991; E:652]

26 The falx cerebri is a sickle-shaped double fold of the inner dura which projects into the longitudinal fissure in the midline between the cerebral hemispheres. Anteriorly, it is narrow and is attached to the crista galli. Posteriorly, it is broad and supports the tentorium cerebelli, as a ridge would a tent. In this posterior region, the straight sinus is found. The fixed margin of the falx cerebri, attached to the skull in the median plane, contains the superior sagittal sinus between its layers. Its free inferior margin contains the inferior sagittal sinus. The falx cerebri protects the brain by preventing excessive side-to-side displacement of the cerebral hemispheres. Because it contains the sinuses, it has a role in the venous drainage of the brain.

The falx cerebelli is a small double fold of the inner dural layer. It lies in the mid-sagittal plane, being attached to the internal occipital crest. Superiorly it is attached to the inferior aspect of the tentorium cerebelli. Its anterior free margin fits into the posterior cerebellar notch. It contains the occipital sinus between its layers. Its function is to help maintain the cerebellum in place.
[A:986; B:599; E:698]

27 The cavernous sinuses lie on either side of the body of the sphenoid bone. They extend from the superior orbital fissure, anteriorly, to the apex of the petrous temporal bone, posteriorly. Numerous fibrous strands, covered with endothelium, cross their lumina. The internal carotid artery passes through the sinus from

posterior to anterior, hugging its medial wall. Its adventitia is separated from the venous blood of the sinus by a layer of endothelium. The artery is surrounded by a plexus of sympathetic nerves. The abducent nerve (VI) passes through the sinus inferior to the internal carotid artery. The lateral wall of the sinus has four nerves embedded in it (running from posterior to anterior). From superior to inferior these are the oculomotor (III), the trochlea (IV), the ophthalmic division of the trigeminal (V_1) and the maxillary division of the trigeminal (V_2). Posteriorly the trigeminal ganglion replaces these last two nerves. It lies in a dural cave (Meckel) on the lateral wall of the sinus.
[A:695; E:698; G:750]

28 The afferent veins of the cavernous sinus are three: first, the superior ophthalmic vein, via the superior orbital fissure, drains the orbit into the anterior part of the cavernous sinus; second, the middle cerebral vein pierces the roof of the sinus; third, the sphenoparietal sinus runs round the lesser wing of the sphenoid and pierces the roof of the sinus. Also draining into the sinus are the inferior ophthalmic vein and central vein of the retina. The efferent veins of the cavernous sinus are the superior petrosal sinus and the inferior petrosal sinus. The sinus also communicates with the pterygoid plexus of veins via the foramen ovale. It should be noted that the cavernous sinuses communicate with each other across the midline.
[A:695; E:705]

29 In the child of 6 months the bones of the vault of the skull are not united by sutures. They are separated by fibrous membranes and, at the corners of the bones, these membranes form large areas called fontanelles. The anterior fontanelle is diamond-shaped and is situated between the two frontal and the two parietal bones. It disappears at about the age of 18 months. The posterior fontanelle is triangular. It lies between the occipital bone, posteriorly, and the two parietal bones, anterolaterally. It is fused by the end of the first year. The fontanelles may be palpated as soft depressions. Together with the interparietal suture, they resemble an arrow, pointing anteriorly. This

has led to the adoption of the word sagittal (arrow-like) to describe this particular anatomical plane. Furthermore, the superior sagittal sinus lies immediately inferior to these fontanelles in the mid-sagittal plane. A needle may be passed through its fibrous roof into this sinus, therefore, for the withdrawal of venous blood from an infant.
[A:310; G:105; H:19]

30 The straight sinus is situated at the junction of the falx cerebri with the tentorium cerebelli. It is formed anteriorly by the confluence of the great cerebral vein (of Galen) and the inferior sagittal sinus. It ends posteriorly by turning laterally to form one of the transverse sinuses, usually the left.
[A:693; B:608]

31 The superior sagittal sinus is situated at the attached border of the falx cerebri. It lies in a space between the two layers of the dura. Thus, superiorly, is the periosteal dura. Inferolaterally are the two layers of the meningeal dura, coming together, inferiorly, to form the falx. The sinus is lined with endothelium. It contains no muscle in its wall and is valveless.
[A:693; C:860]

B Applied answers

32 A lateral plain x-ray of skull is the most valuable to see the size and shape of the hypophyseal fossa. A tumour of the pituitary gland may cause erosion of the clinoid processes and be seen enlarging the bony fossa in all directions.
[I:268; J:16]

33 Thrombosis of the superior sagittal dural venous sinus will cause blockage in the normal flow of CSF, as most of this fluid drains via the arachnoid granulations into this sinus. Reduced drainage with continuing production of CSF will cause the pressure to rise rapidly, and within a day or so the patient may become comatose. The treatment is simply to drain off the excess fluid by repeated lumbar punctures until the venous sinus recanalises itself.
[G:724; H:61; J:134]

34 The arcuate eminence of the petrous temporal bone is caused by the underlying superior semicircular canal of the inner ear.
[I:321; J:28]

35 The nerve of the pterygoid canal consists of fibres from both the greater superficial petrosal and the deep petrosal nerves. The deep petrosal carries sympathetic postganglionic fibres, which lie around the internal carotid artery as a plexus, and enter the skull through the carotid canal. The greater petrosal nerve carries preganglionic parasympathetic fibres which synapse in the pterygopalatine ganglion before supplying the lacrimal gland via the zygomatic and lacrimal nerves. It is also secretory to the mucosal glands of the nasal cavity and palate. A most important component of the greater petrosal nerve is taste fibres from the palate which pass through the pterygopalatine ganglion, on their way to the cell bodies in the geniculate ganglion. The consequences of damage to all these fibres in the pterygoid canal would result in dryness of the nose and palate, reduced tear formation and loss of taste from the palate.
[G:7159; H:48]

36 The tegmen tympani of the adult is a thin sheet of compact bone separating the cranial cavity above from the tympanic cavity below. Because the middle ear and mastoid air cells are a fairly common site of infection, it is an important wall of resistance to brain abscess formation. In the young, the unossified petrosquamous suture is prone to allow direct spread from the middle ear to the cranial meninges.
[G:779; H:28]

37 The cribriform plate is so called due to its numerous sieve-like (L. *cribrum* = sieve) holes on each side of the crista galli. It is through these tiny holes that the olfactory nerve fibres pass to the upper epithelium of the nasal cavity and, hence, how one detects smells. Any fracture here will slice the fragile olfactory nerve fibres as they pierce the horizontal plate of the ethmoid bone. Because the olfactory nerve is not a true cranial nerve but is essentially a direct cerebral outgrowth, it is covered with the three meninges. Consequently, if the meninges are

torn, CSF will leak down the nose. It can be distinguished from a normal runny nose by the increased glucose content of the discharge.
[G:7131; H:31]

38 By using the anterior fontanelle, which is open at this age. The needle is introduced at the lateral edge of this diamond-shaped area between the membranous portions of the frontal and parietal bones. Advanced vertically to the skin, it will soon pierce the dura mater and enter the subdural layer where the haematoma is situated. In the young infant the presence of fontanelles makes burr-holes unnecessary.
[H:19]

39 Some of the veins on the face, especially the region around the eyes and deep tissues of the cheek, drain via the ophthalmic veins and pterygoid venous plexus into the cavernous dural venous sinus. This lies each side of the pituitary gland and contains within its walls cranial nerves III, IV, V and VI on their way to the eye. Consequently, pus on the cheek, if pressed into the veins draining towards the cavernous sinus, may precipitate an abscess, causing cavernous sinus thrombosis. This in turn will lead to pressure of the VIth nerve and a lateral rectus palsy may be the result.
[D:323; G:749; H:43]

40 The dural venous sinuses are best seen as the late stages of either a carotid or a vertebral arteriogram. About four seconds following its injection, the contrast medium may be seen in the major veins and venous sinuses. They may be viewed in the standard anteroposterior and lateral views, the latter being easier for the inexperienced viewer to comprehend.
[I:471; J:134]

C Information answers

41 Both the dartos muscle and the platysma are situated in the superficial fascia. The similarity ends there, however, because the dartos is innervated by the autonomic nervous system,

and the platysma by voluntary nerves; viz. the cervical branch of the facial nerve.
[A:504, 519; G:93, 215]

42 The skin over the angle of the jaw is supplied by the great auricular nerve (C2, 3), a branch of the cervical plexus. Its territory is marked posteriorly by the anterior border of sternomastoid. Behind this line the skin is supplied by the lesser occipital nerve (C2), also a branch of the cervical plexus. Anterior to the parotid, the skin of the face is supplied by the trigeminal nerve.
[A:1035; H:35]

43 The skin of the 'moustache' area of the upper lip is supplied by the infraorbital branch of the trigeminal nerve. It is a branch of the nerve of the maxillary process in development. The central area of the upper lip, philtrum, belongs to the frontonasal process which, in development, is supplied by the ophthalmic division of the trigeminal. However, as development proceeds, this area is 'taken over' by the maxillary nerve. In cases of non-fusion of the frontonasal and maxillary processes (hare-lip), the philtrum retains its ancient nerve supply.
[A:120, 1009; D:291]

44 The muscles of facial expression are conveniently divided into sphincters and dilators. All are supplied by the facial nerve. The sphincters surround the eyelids and the mouth. They are termed orbicularis oculi and orbicularis oris, respectively.
[A:496; H:34]

45 The scalp consists of five layers. Most superficial is the skin. Below this is a layer of fibrofatty connective tissue, the septa of which unite the skin to the next deepest layer—the aponeurosis of the occipitofrontalis muscle (galea aponeurotica). Below the aponeurosis is a layer of loose areolar tissue which separates it from the pericranium (periosteum) of the skull. It is through this loose areolar layer that the layers of the scalp become separated in scalping. The layers of the scalp may be easily

memorised as the letters SCALP stand for each layer in turn

S   skin
C   connective tissue
A   aponeurosis
L   loose connective tissue
P   periosteum

[A:497; D:332; E:651]

46   The arterial supply of the scalp is plentiful and there are free anastomoses between the individual arteries. The arteries on each side (from anterior to posterior) are the supratrochlear, the supraorbital, the superficial temporal, the posterior auricular and the occipital. The supraorbital and supratrochlear are branches of the ophthalmic artery, which accompany the corresponding nerves. The ophthalmic artery arises from the internal carotid. The superficial temporal, posterior auricular and occipital arteries are all branches of the external carotid. The superficial temporal artery accompanies the auriculotemporal nerve.

[A:497, 628, 635; G:719]

47   The secretomotor supply to the parotid gland is via the parasympathetic system. The preganglionic pathway commences at the inferior salivary nucleus and leaves the brain in the glossopharyngeal nerve. The nerve fibres leave the glossopharyngeal nerve in its tympanic branch and pass through the floor of the tympanic cavity to the middle ear. Here they disperse to form the tympanic plexus but are reassembled as the lesser superficial petrosal nerve. This nerve runs in a groove on the petrous temporal bone under the dura of the middle cranial fossa. It leaves the cranium via the foramen ovale to reach the otic ganglion immediately below. Here the parasympathetic secretomotor fibres synapse. The postganglionic fibres are distributed to the gland via the auriculotemporal branch of the mandibular nerve.

[A:1019, 1067; B:672; E:738]

48   From lateral to medial, the structures which lie within the parotid gland are: the facial nerve, the retromandibular vein and the external carotid artery. The facial nerve leaves the skull via the stylomastoid foramen and enters the poster-

ior part of the gland. As it runs forwards, within the gland, it breaks up into its five terminal branches. Deep to the facial nerve is the retromandibular vein. Its plane splits the gland into superficial and deep areas. It is formed by the union of the maxillary and superficial temporal veins, and runs superoinferiorly. As it leaves the inferior aspect of the gland, it divides into anterior and posterior divisions. Deep to the retromandibular vein is the external carotid artery. It runs inferosuperiorly. At the level of the neck of the mandible, it divides into its two terminal branches: the superficial temporal and the maxillary arteries.

[A:1209; E:666; G:716; H:34]

C Applied answers

49 The orbicularis oculi muscle is the sphincter of the palpebral fissure. It consists of an inner palpebral portion, within the lids, and an outer orbital portion, which comprises a complete ring and is attached only to the medial palpebral ligament. This attachment means that upon contraction of the muscle, as in blinking, tears are forced from the lateral aspect of the palpebral fissure, where they are secreted by the lacrimal gland, towards the medial aspect, where they drain via the lacrimal puncta. Damage causes the lower lid to fall away from the eye (ectropion). A stagnant pool of tears will then form in the lower fornix, which will eventually spill over the paralysed lower lid. Infection may occur in this pool, and the resulting conjunctivitis will increase the secretion of tears with further weeping. Paralysis of the orbicularis oculi will result in lack of protection of the cornea, which will also dry out and subsequently may ulcerate.

[E:716; F:457; G:752; J:274]

50 Herpes zoster tends to map out dermatomes. In this case we are dealing with the distribution from the infraorbital, zygomaticofacial and zygomaticotemporal nerves, these being the terminal sensory branches of the maxillary nerve. The area of distribution is developmentally the maxillary process, and consists of the skin of the cheek below the eye and above the upper

lip, but not including the nose or philtrum because these develop from the frontonasal process and are therefore supplied by the ophthalmic nerve. The maxillary region also includes a small area superolateral to the eye, so the overall supply is a wing-shaped area. It is bounded above by branches of the ophthalmic and below by branches of the mandibular divisions of the trigeminal nerve.
[D:289; E:655; G:718]

51 The sphincters of the face (i.e. orbicularis oris and the two orbiculares oculi) are the most important facial muscles. Not only do they contribute to expression but they are also the anchors into which the majority of the other small facial muscles attach. Orbicularis oculi is the protector of the cornea and is therefore necessary for normal vision. Loss of orbicularis oris may lead to a mouth which drools uncontrollably, and is commonly seen in a facial nerve palsy (Bell).
[E:622; G:717; H:34]

52 The vestibule is the area between the cheek and teeth which is normally cleared of food by the actions of buccinator muscle and the tongue. A VIIth cranial nerve lesion will result in paralysis of this muscle and consequent collection of food within the vestibule. It will also lead to drooling from the corner of the mouth.
[E:681; G:780]

53 A lesion of V_1 will result in the cornea being insensitive to touch and so specks of dust or grit will not be felt in the eye. This quickly leads to corneal ulceration and scarring, which if not controlled may cause blindness. It is for this reason that after anaesthetising an eye it is most important to cover the patient's eye or he may collect more foreign bodies than he started with when coming to the surgery!
[E:727; F:499; H:56]

54 Collections of pus in the scalp tend to lie below the aponeurosis in the layer of loose areolar connective tissue but, due to the attachments of the occipitofrontalis, the abscess cannot track laterally. Fluid lying below the muscle layer

can, however, track anteriorly to form an orbital haematoma.
[D:332; E:652; G:722]

55 It is through the loose areolar tissue layer which a person is scalped.
[D:332; E:652; G:722]

56 A generalised scalp infection will drain to the horizontal group of lymph nodes, which are a ring of nodes lying along the superior limits of the cervical investing fascia. These are the sub-mandibular, buccal, parotid, mastoid and occi-pital nodes. The majority of these groups of lymph nodes eventually drain into the chain of deep cervical nodes which are situated along the internal jugular vein.
[D:326; E:650; G:913]

57 The valveless emissary veins connect the di-ploic veins of the cranium with the superficial veins of the scalp. The diploic veins are in direct continuity with the dural venous sinuses, and therefore an abscess on the scalp may well pass infection into an intracranial sinus, thus form-ing a brain abscess.
[E:652; G:720; H:29]

58 Mumps is a viral inflammation of the parotid gland and this in itself is enough to cause pain. However, swelling of the parotid gland is made even more painful by the anatomical fact that the deep investing cervical (polo-neck) fascia splits around the gland and thus swelling causes tension within this restricted fascial plane. Movements of the inflamed fascia such as opening the jaw or yawning increase the tension and result in further pain.
[E:623]

59 The VIIth cranial nerve (facial) exits the skull through the stylomastoid foramen and turns anteriorly to pass right through the substance of the parotid gland, where it splits into its five main branches. It is here likened to a goose's foot (pes anserinus) and any tumour of the parotid gland may easily involve one or more branches which supply the muscles of facial expression.
[G:767; H:35]

60 It depends where the cut is performed, as it is along the auriculotemporal nerve that the postganglionic parasympathetic secretomotor fibres reach the parotid gland from the otic ganglion. If it is made high up on the temporal region, a lesion of the auriculotemporal nerve will only cause loss of scalp sensation; if it is made deep in the temporal fossa, proximal to its parotid branches, it will cause a loss of parotid secretions.
[E:670; G:767; H:34]

61 The opening of the parotid duct (Stensen) is in the vestibule above the second upper molar tooth. To palpate the duct, ask your patient to clench his teeth and the duct can be easily rolled on the contracted masseter muscle just a finger's breadth below and parallel to the zygomatic arch.
[E:666; G:767; H:35; J:230]

D Information answers

62 The middle meningeal artery is encircled by the two roots of the auriculotemporal nerve. This nerve is a branch of the posterior division of the mandibular part of V. It runs deep to the neck of the mandible and then turns upwards between the external auditory meatus and the temporomandibular joint. The nerve is sensory to the skin of the auricle, external auditory meatus, tympanic membrane and that skin overlying the parotid and temporal aspect of the scalp. It carries postganglionic parasympathetic fibres from the otic ganglion to the parotid gland.
[A:1007; E:670]

63 The facial nerve gives off a branch within the petrous temporal bone at the level of the geniculate ganglion. This is the greater superficial petrosal nerve, and it contains preganglionic parasympathetic fibres destined for the sphenopalatine ganglion. It runs forwards in a groove in the petrous temporal bone, immediately deep to the dura of the middle cranial fossa, to reach the foramen lacerum. Here it is joined by the deep petrosal nerve. The deep petrosal nerve is a branch of the sympathetic plexus

surrounding the internal carotid artery. The parasympathetic and sympathetic elements fuse to form the nerve of the pterygoid canal (Vidian nerve). This enters the pterygoid canal, which is a bony tunnel situated at the base of the pterygoid process of the sphenoid and running anteriorly through it to the pterygopalatine fossa. Here the nerve enters the sphenopalatine ganglion and the parasympathetic elements synapse. Postganglionic fibres are distributed to the lacrimal and nasal glands.
[A:1012; G:87, 7163; H:49]

64　The middle meningeal artery arises from the first part of the maxillary artery. It runs upwards, superficial to the sphenomandibular ligament and deep to the lateral pterygoid muscle. It passes between the two roots of the auriculotemporal nerve to enter the skull via the foramen spinosum. Within the skull it divides into anterior and posterior divisions on the squamous temporal bone near the pterion, an important surface marking. The anterior branch crosses the greater wing of the sphenoid to lie on the parietal bone where it runs adjacent to the precentral (motor) sulcus. The posterior branch runs onto the posterior aspect of the parietal bone. Both branches supply bone and meninges.
[A:629; G:724; H:54]

65　The lateral pterygoid arises by two heads. The upper head arises from the infratemporal surface of the greater wing of the sphenoid, the lower head from the lateral aspect of the lateral pterygoid plate. The fibres run backwards and converge to form a tendon, which is inserted into the anterior aspect of the neck of the mandible and into the articular disc of the temporomandibular joint. Contraction of this muscle pulls the combined mandible and disc forwards (protrusion of the jaw). The head of the mandible leaves the articular fossa and comes to lie on the articular eminence as this anterior movement proceeds. Protrusion of the jaw is a necessary accompaniment to opening the mouth (depression of the jaw). If it did not occur, the angle of the jaw would press on the parotid gland and associated structures every time the mouth was opened.
[A:502; E:676; H:38]

66   The temporomandibular joint is a synovial joint
     of the condylar variety. The bones involved are
     the articular fossa and the eminence of the
     temporal bone and the head of the mandible. A
     fibrocartilaginous disc is interposed between
     these bones and is intimately connected to the
     tendon of the lateral pterygoid muscle. The
     joint is unusual in that both articular surfaces
     are covered in fibrocartilage instead of the usual
     hyaline variety.
     [A:407; E:673; G:770]

67   At the temporomandibular joint the mandible
     may be depressed or elevated, protruded or
     retracted. Depression is a simple hinge
     movement between the head of the mandible
     and the combined disc and articular fossa. It is
     brought about by the contraction of the digas-
     trics, geniohyoids and mylohyoids. It is always
     associated with protrusion, in order to prevent
     the angle of the mandible pressing upon poster-
     ior relations. Elevation, the opposite of depres-
     sion, is a powerful movement brought about by
     the temporales, masseters and medial ptery-
     goids. Protrusion of the mandible is a
     movement whereby the head of the mandible
     plus the disc are pulled bodily forwards onto
     the articular eminence. It is brought about by
     the lateral pterygoids. The reverse action is
     retraction. This is performed by the posterior
     fibres of temporalis.
     [A:407; B:665; C:836; F:531]

68   The pterygoid hamulus is a small hook of bone
     at the inferior aspect of the medial pterygoid
     plate. The pterygomandibular raphe attaches to
     it and separates the buccinator muscle anter-
     iorly from the superior constrictor muscle of the
     pharynx posteriorly. The extreme upper part of
     the superior constrictor attaches to the hamu-
     lus. The tendon of the tensor palati winds
     round the hamulus from lateral to medial, to
     reach the palate. A bursa intervenes between
     the tendon and the bone.
     [A:290; G:7112]

69   The pterygomandibular raphe stretches be-
     tween the hamulus of the medial pterygoid
     plate superiorly and the posterior end of the
     mylohyoid line of the mandible inferiorly. It is

merely the fibrous junction of two muscles: the buccinator anteriorly and the superior constrictor posteriorly.
[A:500; E:674; G:955]

D Applied answers

70 The artery involved in extradural bleeding and haematomata formation is the middle meningeal artery. The pterion is a useful surface marking for it, as the artery enters the skull through the foramen spinosum in the sphenoid bone. The middle meningeal artery, a branch of the maxillary artery, is often encircled by the auriculotemporal nerve.
[E:614; G:781; H:54; J:172]

71 The pterygoid venous plexus, which lies deep within the temporal fossa surrounding the lateral pterygoid muscle, is connected with both the ophthalmic and the anterior facial veins. Thus the plexus drains into the cavernous sinus, and so pus within this venous plexus may cause direct increased ophthalmic venous pressure or may even lead to a cavernous sinus thrombosis with resultant paralysis of extra-ocular muscles.
[E:673; H:43]

72 The mastoid process is little developed at birth, as the air sacs are still rudimentary and consequently the facial nerve is very exposed as it exits the stylomastoid foramen. It can be palpated in the newborn and it is not surprising that, if trapped beneath forceps during delivery, a temporary facial palsy may result.
[G:1010]

73 The parotid duct lies a finger's breadth below and parallel to the zygomatic arch; it can be rolled on a tensed masseter, particularly along its anterior border before it pierces the buccinator muscle.
[D:309; E:666; G:767]

74 To perform an inferior dental block, the dentist must place the anaesthetic agent around the inferior alveolar (dental) nerve. This is usually performed just above the lingula of the mand-

ible, which protects the mandibular foramen through which the nerve enters the bone. Due to the proximity of the other major sensory branch of the mandibular division of V, the lingual nerve, it is also not uncommon to cause numbness of the tongue.
[E:669; F:574; G:781]

75 The pterygopalatine (sphenopalatine) ganglion, which lies in the pterygopalatine fossa, is the largest peripheral ganglion of the parasympathetic system. If stimulated, it simulates 'hay fever', causing streaming of the eyes, running of the nose and mucous secretions from the palate. The preganglionic fibres reach the ganglion by way of the facial nerve and the greater superficial petrosal nerve. The postganglionic fibres are then distributed along the zygomaticotemporal, lacrimal, palatine and nasal nerves to the lacrimal gland and mucous glands of the palate and nose.
[F:568; G:745; H:49]

76 Lateral views of the temporomandibular joint with the mouth open and closed reveal the articular tubercle and its relationship to the condyloid process (head) of the mandible. The external auditory meatus is also well shown in both these views, with the tympanic plate lying at its inferior margin, protecting it from the mandibular fossa and joint itself.
[I:279; J:26]

77 Boring lectures cause yawning amongst the audience, and yawning is a common cause of jaw dislocation. The lateral pterygoid muscles protrude and depress the jaw. If the other muscles of mastication are relaxed, the head of the mandible may 'click' over the articular tubercle and dislocate anteriorly to lie just alongside the zygomatic arch.
[D:342; E:676]

78 Trismus is a painful tonic spasm of the jaw muscles as seen in diseases such as tetanus (lockjaw). The muscles involved are the medial and lateral pterygoids, temporalis and, above all, the masseter muscle.
[E:666; G:770]

79   The orbit is a four-sided pyramidal-shaped cavity, with its base anteriorly and its apex posteriorly. The orbital margin is divided equally between three bones: superiorly, the frontal bone; anteromedially, the maxilla; and laterally, the zygoma. The roof is formed by the orbital plate of the frontal bone. The medial wall is made up, from anterior to posterior, of the frontal process of the maxilla, the lacrimal bone, the ethmoid and the body of the sphenoid. It is exceedingly thin. The floor is composed of the orbital plate of the maxilla. The lateral wall is made up of the zygomatic bone anteriorly and the greater wing of the sphenoid posteriorly.
[A:262, E:719, H:18]

80   The superior orbital fissure connects the middle cranial fossa with the orbit. It transmits the motor nerves to the muscles of the eyeball (oculomotor nerve III, trochlear nerve IV, abducent nerve VI) and the three branches of the ophthalmic division of the sensory trigeminal nerve (V_1)—the lacrimal nerve, the frontal nerve and the nasociliary nerve. Sympathetic fibres also gain access to the orbit via the superior orbital fissure. The inferior orbital fissure connects the pterygopalatine fossa with the orbit. It transmits two branches of the maxillary division of the trigeminal nerve (V_2): the infraorbital nerve and the zygomatic nerve.
[A:263, 290; B:629; C:897]

81   Tenon's capsule surrounds the eyeball from the optic nerve as far anteriorly as the corneoscleral junction, and separating it from the orbital fat gives it a smooth surface on which to move. The tendons of the six ocular muscles pierce this sheath, the sheath being reflected on them as a tubal covering. The inferior part of the sheath, which passes under the eye, is thickened. It suspends the eye as if it were a sailor in a hammock, and is termed the suspensory ligament of the eye. The suspensory ligament is attached to the lateral and medial walls of the orbit. Their attachments are common to those of the lateral and medial check ligaments, which are prolongations of the tubal

coverings of the lateral and medial recti to the orbital walls.
[A:1128; E:725]

82   The tendinous ring is the origin of the four rectus muscles of the eye. Each arises from its respective part of the ring. The lateral rectus arises by two heads which fuse as they approach the eyeball.
[A:1122; E:719; G:757]

83   The cornea is the major refracting surface of the eyeball, the lens being used for fine adjustment. It is transparent and has no blood supply.
[A:1098; G:765]

84   The four recti (medial, lateral, superior and inferior) arise from their respective sides of the tendinous ring, and diverging are inserted into the corresponding regions of the sclera some 5 mm behind the corneoscleral junction. The medial rectus muscle is a pure adductor and the lateral rectus a pure abductor. However, the muscles are arranged around the plane of the orbital cones, which are not parallel but diverge as they pass anteriorly, and not around the planes of movement of the eyeball. This means that the superior and inferior rectus muscles pass medial to the vertical axis of the eyeball's rotation and act as adductors. Thus the action of the superior rectus is to elevate and adduct the eyeball, and that of the inferior rectus is to depress and adduct it.
     The two oblique muscles counteract the adducting tendency of the superior and inferior recti. The superior oblique muscle arises from the body of the sphenoid superomedial to the tendinous ring. As it passes anteriorly it becomes tendinous. The tendon is slung from a pulley (or trochlea) on the anteromedial wall of the orbit and is inserted into the top of the eyeball. Its action is to turn the eye downwards and outwards (depression and abduction). The inferior oblique arises from the anteromedial part of the orbital floor and passes posterolaterally, to be inserted into the lateral aspect of the eyeball. Its action is to elevate and abduct the eye so that it looks upwards and laterally.
[A:1122; B:636; G:760]

81

85 The muscles of the iris consist of circular fibres and radial fibres. The circular fibres constrict the pupil. They are supplied by parasympathetic nerves which run in the oculomotor nerve, synapse in the ciliary ganglion and pass to the eye in the short ciliary nerves. The radial fibres dilate the pupil. They are supplied by sympathetic fibres which, having already synapsed in the superior cervical ganglion, pass to the internal carotid plexus and from there to the ciliary ganglion. Then they pass 'non-stop' through the ganglion to the eyeball, via the short ciliary nerves. Some sympathetic fibres pass from the nasociliary nerve to its long ciliary branches and thus to the eyeball. These latter sympathetic fibres reached the trigeminal nerve by passing to it from the internal carotid plexus in the cavernous sinus.
[A:1105; B:646; C:194]

86 The optic nerve is accompanied along its entire course by sheaths of dura, arachnoid and pia. The meninges eventually fuse with the sclera of the eyeball. It is therefore surrounded by the subarachnoid space along its entire course. Cranial nerves possess no such prolongation of the subarachnoid space, the dura fusing with the perineurium soon after their origin. The optic nerve should therefore be regarded as a diverticulum of the brain and not a true cranial nerve.
[A:997; E:725]

87 The ciliary ganglion is situated in the posterior portion of the orbit, immediately lateral to the optic nerve. It contains the synapses for parasympathetic nerves passing to the intrinsic muscles of the eyeball.
[A:999; H:56]

88 The ciliary ganglion is a parasympathetic ganglion. It receives preganglionic fibres from the oculomotor nerve via the branch to the inferior oblique muscle. In the ganglion the fibres synapse. Postganglionic fibres run to the eyeball via the 12 short ciliary nerves. They supply the ciliary muscle and the circular fibres of the iris (sphincter pupillae).
[A:999; H:56]

89 Both the long and short ciliary nerves contain sensory fibres. However, the long ciliary nerves also contain sympathetic fibres destined for the dilator pupillae. The short ciliary nerves contain both sympathetic and parasympathetic fibres for the dilator and sphincter pupillae, respectively.
[A:1003; G:754; H:56]

E Applied answers

90 A stye is an infection of a sebaceous gland situated at the base of the eyelash. A Meibomian cyst is due to a blocked tarsal gland which lies just posterior to the eyelash within the lids. These glands secrete an oily material which readily forms a noticeable cystic swelling if their drainage is impaired. These cysts often go unnoticed until infected, when they may easily be confused with a stye.
[E:716; G:761]

91 Ptosis may be congenital but there are two anatomical causes due to the two different muscles involved in keeping the upper eyelid raised. The greater portion of muscle fibres are the voluntary fibres of levator palpebrae superioris but the smooth muscle fibres of the superior tarsal muscle also contribute to the normal width of the palpebral fissure. The voluntary muscle is innervated by the IIIrd cranial nerve whilst the smooth muscle is controlled by sympathetic fibres from the superior cervical ganglion. Damage to either of these nerves will cause ptosis.
[E:720; F:495; G:753]

92 Papilloedema is caused by an increase in CSF pressure. The reason why it can be readily seen at the optic disc is that the optic nerve is not a true cranial nerve but a brain extension and is therefore surrounded by the three meninges. A rise in intracranial pressure will be transmitted therefore along the subarachnoid space and seen on the retina as swelling of the optic disc.
[E:725; F:503; G:731]

93 To test accommodation, your patient looks into the distance and is then asked to focus on a near

object such as a pin. Three things happen: the eyes focus, the pupils constrict and the eyes converge. The pupillary and focusing changes are through afferent connections of the optic nerve with the pretectal area and efferent preganglionic parasympathetic neurons from the Edinger–Westphal nucleus. These efferent fibres, carried by the IIIrd cranial nerve, synapse in the ciliary ganglion and the postganglionic fibres pass to the ciliary and constrictor pupillae muscles.
[B:646; D:385; F:499]

94 Central artery thrombosis causes instant blindness, as this is the only arterial supply to the retina and is a classic example of an 'end-artery'. The central retinal artery is easily seen on ophthalmoscopy, as it leaves the protection of the optic nerve at the disc and divides into its temporal and nasal branches which supply the retina in a quadrantic manner.
[B:649; D:410; F:503]

95 The ptosis is likely to be due to sympathetic or IIIrd cranial nerve problems. The dilated pupil may be due to loss of parasympathetic control, and the position of the eyeball indicates a loss of those muscles supplied by the IIIrd cranial nerve (i.e. medial rectus, inferior oblique, superior and inferior recti). All these signs can be explained by damage to the oculomotor nerve (III) and its parasympathetic fibres.
[E:721; F:499; G:764]

96 The integrity of the sympathetic chain must be checked in cases of ptosis. An interruption in the sympathetic outflow from T1 may be caused by tumours in the apex of the lung. These tumours may also involve the brachial plexus and innervation of the hand (Pancoast's tumour).
[D:328; E:28; G:936, 946]

97 The blind spot is where the fibres of the optic nerve pass through the retinal layers. It is the pale area seen on ophthalmoscopy as the optic disc and is of course also the point of entry of the retinal artery. It lies on the nasal side of the fundus.
[B:649; E:725]

98 The normal pressure of the aqueous humour is about 25 mmHg. A blockage in its normal drainage mechanism may cause acute glaucoma. Secreted by the ciliary body, the aqueous humour flows from posterior to anterior chambers before draining at the lateral angle of the iris into the corneoscleral junction, where lies an endothelial-lined canal (Schlemm). The fluid drains across the endothelial lining and into the ocular veins. This canal is so situated that prolonged dilatation of the pupil may cause an impedance to the flow of aqueous humour in some people who possess a particularly shallow anterior chamber, due to bunching of the iris against its opening.
[B:644; F:502; G:765]

99 This is a VIth cranial nerve palsy affecting the lateral rectus muscle, its only motor supply. Due to the intracranial length of this slender nerve, the condition of lateral rectus palsy may be caused by increased intracranial pressure from whatever origin.
[G:740; H:56]

F Information answers

100 The nasal septum consists of the perpendicular plate of the ethmoid superiorly, the vomer posteroinferiorly and the septal cartilage anteriorly.
[A:278, 1088; D:403; G:7108]

101 The functions of the nasal cavity can be subdivided into those concerned with respiration and those concerned with olfaction. The respiratory mucous membrane covering the lower part of the nasal cavity has a rich blood supply. This serves to warm and moisten the inhaled air. The mucus secreted by this epithelium traps large particles such as dust, which is wafted to the pharynx by cilia and then swallowed. The olfactory mucous membrane lines the sphenoethmoidal recess and the upper part of the superior concha and adjacent septum. It contains the nerve endings of the olfactory nerves. For the detection of smell, the substances involved must be in solution. This area is therefore supplied with numerous serous glands.

The paranasal air sinuses lighten the skull. They are supposed to impart a resonant quality to the voice in rather the same way as a soundbox does in a stringed instrument.
[A:278, 1087; G:7109; H:55]

102 The lateral wall of the nose is divided up by three projections: the superior, middle and inferior conchae. Above the superior concha is the sphenoethmoidal recess. Between the conchae are the superior and middle meati. Below the inferior concha is the inferior meatus. The sphenoidal air sinuses open into the sphenoethmoidal recess. The posterior cells of the ethmoidal sinus enter into the superior meatus. The middle meatus has a prominence on it—the bulla ethmoidalis, caused by the underlying middle ethmoidal cells. The middle ethmoidal cells open on its superior aspect. Below the bulla is a semicircular furrow—the hiatus semilunaris.

The anterior ethmoidal cells, and their continuation, the frontal sinuses, open into the anterior aspect of the hiatus. The maxillary sinus opens into the posterior aspect. Infection may easily spread therefore from frontal sinuses to maxillary sinuses via the hiatus semilunaris.

The inferior meatus receives the nasolacrimal duct guarded by a valve of mucous membrane. This prevents air being blown in a retrograde manner up the duct.
[A:278, 1087; E:755; G:7115; H:31]

103 Five arteries anastomose on the anteroinferior part of the nasal septum. This region is termed 'Little's area' and is a frequent source of epistaxis. The arteries are, first, the septal branch of the sphenopalatine artery, which is in turn derived from the maxillary. It enters the nose posteriorly from the pterygopalatine fossa via the sphenopalatine foramen. Second and third are the anterior ethmoidal and posterior ethmoidal arteries, both branches of the ophthalmic. They leave the orbit via foramina in its medial wall. Fourth is the great palatine artery, a branch of the maxillary. This artery reaches the nose via the incisive foramen in the palate. Last is the septal branch of the superior labial artery, which is in turn a branch of the facial artery.
[A:1092; G:7111]

104 The hard palate is supplied with sensory nerves from the maxillary division of the trigeminal via the pterygopalatine ganglion. These nerves are the greater palatine, the lesser palatine and the nasopalatine. The greater and lesser palatine nerves descend in the palatine canal and, passing through the palatine foramen, appear on the inferior surface of the back of the hard palate. The greater palatine nerves pass anteriorly. The lesser palatine nerves pass posteriorly and onto the anterior aspect of the soft palate. The nasopalatine nerves descend on the vomer and pass through the incisive canal onto the anterior part of the hard palate.

The soft palate is supplied by the pharyngeal plexus. This is derived from the glossopharyngeal nerves, vagus nerves and sympathetic system. The glossopharyngeal nerve supplies the soft palate with sensory fibres. The muscles of the soft palate are supplied by the vagus (or, more correctly, the accessory nerve), except tensor palati which is supplied by the trigeminal nerve (mandibular division).
[A:1006, 1007, 1011; E:749; G:86, 748, 7109]

105 The palatine tonsils are aggregates of lymphoid tissue situated at the posterolateral aspect of the oral cavity. Each tonsil lies between the palatoglossal arch anteriorly and the palatopharyngeal arch posteriorly. It lies on some loose areolar tissue which separates it from the superior constrictor of the pharynx. Superior to the tonsil is the soft palate; inferiorly, the posterior part of the tongue. The tonsil is largely supplied with blood by the tonsillar artery, a branch of the facial artery, which is situated immediately deep to the superior constrictor.
[A:1244; D:299; E:749; G:962; H:47]

106 Waldeyer's ring comprises the nasopharyngeal adenoids, the palatine tonsils and the aggregates of lymphoid tissue on the dorsum of the tongue (lingual tonsil). Together they comprise a complete ring of lymphoid tissue surrounding the oronasal aperture of the body.
[A:1238, 1244; G:957; H:47]

107 The pterygopalatine ganglion (sphenopalatine ganglion) is situated in the pterygopalatine fossa and is suspended from the maxillary

nerve. It is comprised of three roots: parasympathetic, sympathetic and sensory. Only the parasympathetic fibres synapse in the ganglion; the rest pass straight through.

The parasympathetic fibres originate in the facial nerve but leave it in the petrous temporal bone as the greater superficial petrosal nerve. This unites at the foramen lacerum with the sympathetic greater petrosal nerve, to form the nerve of the pterygoid canal. Passing through the pterygoid canal, both sets of fibres reach the ganglion. Having synapsed, the parasympathetic fibres are distributed to the glands of the nose and pharynx and to the lacrimal gland via the zygomatic nerve. They are secretomotor to these glands.

The sympathetic root is comprised of the sympathetic fibres of the greater petrosal nerve. They are postganglionic, having already synapsed in the superior cervical ganglion.

Fibres from the maxillary nerve form the sensory root. They pass straight through the ganglion and form the bulk of its branches.
[A:1005; F:558; G:745, 794]

108 There are three constrictor muscles in the pharynx—superior, middle and inferior. The lowest fibres of the superior constrictor are overlapped by the upper fibres of the middle constrictor. Similarly, the upper fibres of the inferior constrictor overlap the lower fibres of the middle constrictor. The musculature of the pharynx therefore resembles three straight beer glasses (or flowerpots, for those horticulturally minded), placed one inside the other.
[A:1246; G:952; H:50]

109 The inferior constrictor consists of two parts. The upper part arises from the oblique line on the thyroid cartilage. The fibres pass backwards to be inserted into the midline posterior pharyngeal raphe. It is sometimes termed the thyropharyngeus.

The lower part arises from the cricoid cartilage and forms a ring of muscle. It acts as a sphincter for the upper end of the oesophagus and, indeed, its fibres blend with those of the oesophagus. It is sometimes called cricopharyngeus. A potential weakness is present between these two portions of the inferior constrictor

called Killian's dehiscence. It is here that pharyngeal diverticulae may develop.
[A:1246; D:302; F:555; G:959]

110 The pharyngeal plexus is derived from branches of the glossopharyngeal nerve, the sympathetic system and the vagus nerve (strictly, the accessory). It supplies all the muscles of the pharynx and soft palate except stylopharyngeus, which is supplied from the glossopharyngeal direct, and the tensor palati, which is supplied by the mandibular division of the trigeminal. The musculature of the tongue, both intrinsic and extrinsic, is supplied by the hypoglossal nerve, except for palatoglossus which is supplied by the pharyngeal plexus.
[A:1249]

111 The glossopharyngeal nerve supplies one muscle only—the stylopharyngeus. The nerve descends in the neck in the carotid sheath. It then winds round the stylopharyngeus, supplying it as it does so.
[A:1017; G:960]

112 The hyoid bone moves upwards and forwards during deglutition by the contraction of mylohyoid, geniohyoid, digastric and stylohyoid, thus compressing the food bolus between the tongue and the palate. Simultaneously, the wave of contraction spreads backwards from the anterior part of the tongue. As a result of these actions the food bolus is propelled towards the pharynx.
[A:1249; B:749; E:753]

113 The epiglottis is connected to the posterior of the tongue, in the midline, by a fold of mucous membrane—the median glossoepiglottic fold. Two further mucosal folds connect the lateral aspects of the epiglottis with the pharyngeal wall—the lateral glossoepiglottic folds. Between these three folds are two depressions—the valleculae—which are therefore situated between the tongue and epiglottis, on either side of the midline.
[A:1175; C:939; H:52]

F Applied answers

114 In the younger age group the majority of nose bleeds arise from the anterior septal region where

numerous arteries anastomose. These are the anterior and posterior ethmoidal, sphenopalatine and greater palatine arteries as well as the superior labial branch of the facial artery. The bleeding is often due to playing with or picking from the nasal septum and usually comes from this richly vascular area (Little's area, Kiesselbach's area). Bleeding more posteriorly from the territory of the greater palatine artery is often not controlled by simple pressure of nasal packing and may require ligation of the maxillary artery or even the external carotid artery.
[A:1092; G:7111]

115 The drainage of the frontal paranasal air sinus is by gravity to the middle meatus in the lateral wall of nose. Here, just below the bulla ethmoidalis in the hiatus semilunaris, opens the maxillary sinus. In the latter case, the ostium is near the roof of its cavity. It is therefore easy for infection in the frontal sinuses to drain straight down into the maxillary sinus, which has relatively poor drainage. The floor of the maxillary sinus (Highmore) lies adjacent to the roots and alveolar processes of the upper teeth. Pain from infection in the maxillary sinus is thus quite often indistinguishable from that of dental origin.
[E:755; G:7115; H:48]

116 A technique for allowing a good view of the nasopharynx, posterior rhinoscopy is performed by passing an angled mirror through the open mouth and fauces. Normally one would hope to see the posterior nasal septum (vomer) and the conchae in each nasal cavity as well as the tubal swellings guarding the auditory tubes (Eustachian, pharyngotympanic) superolaterally. In the roof, especially in the young child, one may see the pharyngeal tonsils or adenoids.
[B:737; E:755; G:957]

117 The pharyngotympanic or auditory tube equalises pressure in the middle ear, being opened each time one swallows. Its medial two-thirds is cartilaginous whilst its lateral portion is bony in the adult. In the adult it has a downward path to the nasopharynx from the middle ear, thus allowing mucous secretions to drain freely. In children, however, not only is the tube rela-

tively narrow but it also lies almost horizontal, making drainage difficult. Where it opens in the nasopharynx is the pharyngeal tonsil or adenoid, and any enlargement of this lymphoid mass will obstruct the drainage from the tube. Chronic obstruction causes a collection of sticky mucus in the middle ear (glue ear), which is a ready medium for bacterial growth. In children, whose incidence of upper respiratory tract infection is already high, this may be a recurrent clinical problem.
[B:744; E:736; G:7157; H:59]

118 A 'gag' reflex, often provoked by examination of the posterior nasopharynx, is due to stimulation of the glossopharyngeal nerve (IXth cranial). The sensory innervation of the fauces and pharynx are through the IXth nerve but the movements of the pharynx are through the pharyngeal plexus, which has input from IX, X and the cranial portion of XI as well as a sympathetic contribution.
[B:719; G:89, 810]

119 An enlarged pharyngeal tonsil or adenoid is a cause of auditory tube blockage, leading to recurrent ear infections. If particularly large, its removal may improve mucus drainage of the tympanic cavity and thus reduce the number of middle ear infections.
[E:736; G:7157]

120 The jugulodigastric lymph node is normally palpable at the inferior angle of the jaw in acute tonsillitis.
[E:651; H:38]

121 One would suppose that removal of the epiglottis might lead to inhalation of food through an unprotected larynx. In fact this is not so because the purse-string-like action of the aryepiglottic folds is a much more efficient barrier and thus little inconvenience is felt after epiglottic removal, provided the aryepiglottic folds are repaired.
[G:972; H:52]

122 'Hypopharynx' is a clinical term used to describe the laryngopharynx. Malignant tumours of this region are mainly of epithelial origin, and two anatomical sites are particularly easy to

miss. These are the valleculae at the root of the tongue and the piriform fossae which lie on either side of the laryngeal opening. Indirect laryngoscopy is performed through the open mouth and this simple procedure can check the hypopharynx and valleculae, as well as the vocal cords themselves. If the patient produces a high pitched 'ee-ee' the larynx is raised and cords are easily seen. When phonation ceases, the cords abduct to reveal the upper tracheal rings through the rima glottidis.
[D:308; E:762; G:975]

123 A pharyngeal pouch or diverticulum appears between the two parts of the inferior constrictor muscle. The inferior constrictor has a crico-pharyngeal part and a thyropharyngeal portion, the latter fibres being oblique compared with the horizontal cricopharyngeal fibres. Posteriorly between these two is a weakness (Killian's dehiscence) through which a diverti-culum or pouch may bulge. It is seen more commonly on the left and is thought to be due to inco-ordination of the cricopharyngeus muscle with resultant increased intrapharyn-geal pressure.
[D:302; H:50]

124 The classic site for a fish bone to stick is in the piriform fossa or recess. These fossae are the portion of the laryngopharynx lying either side of the laryngeal inlet, and it is down these two channels that food passes, having been de-flected from the larynx by the elevated epi-glottis.
[G:956; J:232]

G Information answers

125 The styloid process, stylohyoid ligament and the upper half of the body of the hyoid bone are remnants of the cartilage of the second pharyn-geal arch. The greater horn and the lower half of the body of the hyoid bone are remnants of the third pharyngeal arch. Thus the hyoid bone is seen to be a hybrid, being derived from two embryological structures. The thyroid cartilage is the remnant of the cartilage of the fourth pharyngeal arch (and maybe the fifth as well).

The cricoid and arytenoids are derived from the sixth arch cartilage. The stylomandibular ligament is merely a fascial condensation between the parotid and submandibular glands. Unlike the sphenomandibular and stylohyoid ligaments, it has no embryological significance.
[A:120, 503; B:579; F:531]

126 The skeleton of the larynx consists of cartilages which are connected by membranes. The thyroid cartilage consists of two plates which meet anteriorly at a sharp angle. It is deficient posteriorly. Its posterior border has prominent cornua superiorly and inferiorly. The cricoid cartilage is signet ring-shaped. It articulates with the inferior cornu of thyroid cartilage. It is narrower anteriorly than posteriorly. The arytenoid cartilages are two small pyramids of cartilage which articulate on the posterosuperior aspect of the cricoid cartilage. They give attachment to the vocal cords and the muscles which move them. Unlike the other cartilages, which are composed of hyaline cartilage, the epiglottis is made up of elastic cartilage. It is leaf-shaped, being broader superiorly than inferiorly. Inferiorly it attaches to the posterior aspect of the front of the thyroid cartilage.
[A:1173; G:965; H:52]

127 There are two sphincteric mechanisms of the larynx, designed to prevent food and fluids from entering the air passages. One mechanism is situated at the laryngeal inlet. A further back-up mechanism is present at the level of the cords. During swallowing, the larynx is pulled bodily upwards. The epiglottis is pushed backwards by the tongue and covers the laryngeal opening. The opening itself is narrowed by the contraction of the aryepiglottic muscles. Thus food passes over a covered and narrowed inlet. Should any food enter the larynx, however, the vocal cords may be adducted, preventing it from passing any further. Should it get past this second sphincter, the cough reflex is used. The cords are adducted and pressure builds up in the airways by muscular contraction. Sudden release of the cords produces an explosive rush of air which, hopefully, carries the offending particle with it to the exterior.
[A:1173; B:757; G:979; H:53]

128   The posterior cricoarytenoid is the most vital
       muscle of the larynx. This is the only muscle
       capable of abducting the vocal cords and,
       hence, allowing air through the larynx. Its para-
       lysis results in severe stridor. It runs from the
       posterior of the cricoid cartilage superolaterally
       to the muscular process of the arytenoid cartil-
       age.
       [A:1179; G:973; H:53]

129   The sensory nerve supply of the larynx may be
       divided by the vocal cords into that part above
       the cords and that part below. The portion
       above the cords is supplied by the internal
       laryngeal branch of the superior laryngeal
       nerve, which is a branch of the vagus. Below
       the cords sensation is provided by the recurrent
       laryngeal branch of the vagus. The recurrent
       laryngeal nerve supplies all the muscles of the
       larynx except for cricothyroid. This is supplied
       by the external laryngeal branch of the superior
       laryngeal nerve.
       [A:1182; E:759; G:964]

130   The two laminae of the thyroid cartilage meet
       anteriorly at the angle. This angle is prominent
       and is referred to as the laryngeal prominence
       (Adam's apple).
       [A:1174; G:965; H:52]

131   The levator glandulae thyroideae is a fibrous
       band which connects the isthmus of the thyroid
       gland to the hyoid bone. It may contain muscle.
       [A:1374; G:935]

132   Three arteries supply the thyroid gland: the
       superior thyroid artery, the inferior thyroid
       artery and the thyroidea ima artery. The thy-
       roidea ima artery is not always present. The
       superior thyroid artery is a branch of the exter-
       nal carotid and runs vertically downwards to
       the upper pole of the gland in company with
       the external laryngeal nerve. The inferior thy-
       roid artery is a branch of the thyrocervical
       trunk, which is in turn a branch of the first part
       of the subclavian artery. It ascends to the back
       of the gland and is usually tortuous. The recur-
       rent laryngeal nerve is an intimate relation of
       this artery and may be anterior or posterior to it
       or even pass through its branches. The thy-

roidea ima is a branch of the aortic arch or the brachiocephalic artery. It ascends to the isthmus of the gland. The venous drainage of the thyroid gland is via the superior, middle and inferior thyroid veins. The superior and middle thyroid veins drain to the internal jugular vein. The inferior thyroid vein drains to the brachiocephalic veins.
[A:1375; D:286; G:963]

133 The anterior triangle of the neck is bounded by the anterior border of the sternomastoid laterally, the mandible superiorly and the midline of the neck anteriorly. The sternomastoid, therefore, is the structure which divides the neck into its anterior and posterior triangles.
[A:631; B:683; G:91]

134 The deep fascia of the neck forms definite sheets, separating one area from another. The prevertebral and investing layers are two of these. The investing layer surrounds the entire neck and lies deep to the superficial fascia. It is attached below to the clavicle and manubrium, and above to the mandible, zygomatic arch, hyoid and base of the skull. It splits to enclose the parotid and submandibular glands and also the trapezius and sternomastoid muscles. The prevertebral layer covers the muscles anterior to the cervical vertebral column, viz. longus cervicis and capitis. It also covers the scalenes and muscles of the back of the neck. Thus it forms the floor of the posterior triangle. Above, it is attached to the skull. Below, it fuses with the anterior longitudinal ligament at about T4. This limits the spread of pus into the inferior mediastinum.
[A:503; E:623]

135 Both the suprahyoid and infrahyoid muscles contract on swallowing, lifting the hyoid bone and larynx. Try it on yourself! The hyoid bone is raised during the first phase of deglutition by the suprahyoid muscles, forcing the food bolus to the back of the mouth. The larynx is lifted during the second phase by the infrahyoid muscles, preventing the influx of food into the airway.
[A:1249; B:749; C:935; E:753]

136 Literally, 'ansa cervicalis' means the loop of the neck. The hypoglossal nerve contains not only hypoglossal fibres but also some fibres from C1.

These leave the nerve in the carotid triangle as the descending branch (descendens hypoglossi). This descending branch joins with a descending branch of C2 and C3 to form a loop—the ansa cervicalis. The ansa supplies the strap muscles of the neck.
[A:1026; E:632; G:915; H:38]

137 The external carotid artery supplies the neck and the outside of the head with blood. The internal carotid artery has no branches outside the skull. The branches of the external carotid artery in the neck are:

Superior thyroid artery
Ascending pharyngeal artery
Lingual artery
Facial artery
Occipital artery
Posterior auricular artery

It ends at the level of the neck of the mandible by dividing into its two terminal branches—the maxillary artery and the superficial temporal artery.
[A:623; G:712; J:172]

G Applied answers

138 In both sexes during early childhood the larynx is similar in dimensions. At puberty the male laryngeal cartilages enlarge considerably whilst those of the female increase only very slightly. This enlargement accounts for the laryngeal prominence of the thyroid cartilage (Adam's apple) being easily seen and felt in the adult male. The deepening of the male adult voice is due to the increased cartilage size, especially in the anteroposterior diameter which is doubled at puberty.
[A:1174; G:965; H:52]

139 The superior bony structure in the laryngeal skeleton is the hyoid. However, quite commonly in the elderly there is true ossification of the thyroid and cricoid cartilages which, with the arytenoids, are developed in hyaline cartilage. This is rarely seen in the young and does not affect the corniculate, cuneiform or the apex of the arytenoid cartilages which all develop in elastic fibrocartilage and cannot therefore

ossify. This feature is particularly well seen on a lateral xeroradiograph of the neck.
[F:585; G:967; H:52; J:38]

140 The hyoid lies at the level of C2–3 vertebral bodies. The isthmus of the thyroid gland lies anterior to second and third tracheal rings (C7–T1) where it is separated from the strap muscles by the pretracheal fascia. The C6 vertebral level is where the larynx becomes the trachea and the pharynx continues as the oesophagus, and is the position anteriorly of the cricoid cartilage.
[D:279; E:616]

141 The structures seen on indirect laryngoscopy are, first, the base of the tongue and lingual surface of the epiglottis and then, by instructing the patient to produce a high pitched 'ee-ee', the vocal cords are brought into view. On ceasing phonation the cords abduct, revealing the upper tracheal rings through the opened rima glottidis. The vestibular folds above the true cords are pink, fleshy folds of mucous membrane compared with the normal pearly white of the vocal cords. Before withdrawing the mirror, the piriform fossae and valleculae are checked for abnormalities.
[B:754; D:308; E:762; G:975; H:53]

142 The external laryngeal nerve supplies the cricothyroid muscle, paralysis of which causes weakness in the voice due to reduced vocal cord tension. It does not normally affect breathing. The recurrent laryngeal nerves supply all the intrinsic laryngeal muscles except for the cricothyroid and thus a bilateral paralysis results in the cords abducting, leaving only a 'glottic chink' through which inadequate air can pass. The patient has only a hoarse whisper and will suffer respiratory distress, possibly requiring a tracheostomy.
[G:972; H:41]

143 This is because the radiologist has asked the patient to say 'ee-ee' to stretch and adduct the cords. On relaxation and in normal quiet respiration the cords should abduct. If a cord is paralysed, abduction will not take place.
[B:755; I:590; J:40]

144 These procedures are performed in order to relieve acute airways obstruction above or at the level of the vocal cords. Laryngotomy is an opening made just above the cricoid cartilage through the cricothyroid ligament and is usually of a very temporary nature. Tracheostomy is a more permanent procedure, often performed by the surgeon, involving an opening into the trachea usually at the level of the second to fourth tracheal rings. In laryngotomy, besides the skin and an occasional anterior jugular vein, the only structure protecting the airway is the cricothyroid ligament itself. In the normal tracheostomy, however, one needs not only to retract the strap muscles of the neck but also to divide the very vascular isthmus of the thyroid. In children this procedure may endanger the left brachiocephalic vein or even the thymus, which often extends above the suprasternal notch. The secret to both procedures is to keep right in the midline.
[D:21; E:791; G:932; H:39]

145 The tortuous course of the inferior thyroid artery is readily seen on an arch aortogram and is due to the fact that on every swallow the thyroid gland ascends a few centimetres and must naturally drag its arterial supply with it. If this artery had no capability to elongate, it would be traumatised.
[G:936; H:191; J:170]

146 Part of the pretracheal fascia forms the sheath of the thyroid gland and can be seen lying between the two sternohyoid muscles when the investing layer of deep cervical fascia has been incised. Superiorly, it is attached to the oblique line of the thyroid cartilage and the arch of the cricoid. Having enclosed the gland, it passes inferiorly to enclose the inferior thyroid veins and then blend with the posterior surface of the pericardium at the bifurcation of the trachea. Thus, when the laryngeal skeleton ascends during swallowing, so must the thyroid gland.
[E:623; G:926, 934; H:39]

147 The very close but variable relationship between the inferior thyroid artery and the recurrent laryngeal nerves in the posterior part of the gland makes thyroid surgery, especially a total

thyroidectomy, a potential risk to normal speech. Prior to operation it is common practice to check that both cords are in working order so that if there is any problem postoperatively one knows at least the origin of the lesion! If there is any preoperative abnormality then the surgeon is especially careful to leave the posterior region of the gland intact.
[D:286; G:937; H:191]

148 Between the first and second pharyngeal pouches a thyroid diverticulum originates during the fourth week of development. This diverticulum elongates caudally, forming the gland and leaving a solid stalk whose site of attachment can be seen as the foramen caecum of the tongue. An epithelial tract may remain from the dorsum of the tongue to the definitive gland (thyroglossal duct) and occasional cystic swelling may occur (thyroglossal cysts). If such a swelling is midline and elevates on protruding the tongue, then a thyroglossal cyst is the most likely diagnosis. These structures may be anywhere between the foramen caecum and the thyroid gland itself.
[A:169; D:288; F:519; G:935]

149 The two pairs of parathyroid glands develop from the third and fourth pharyngeal pouches. The glands from the third pouch usually migrate caudally with the thymus gland, overtaking the glands from the fourth pouch which lie in the fascial sheath in the upper part of the thyroid gland. Variations in number, size and position are common and aberrant third pouch parathyroid glands may descend with the thymus to a retrosternal position instead of the more common site in the inferior lobe of the thyroid gland.
[A:170; D:288; E:646; G:963]

150 The carotid sheath is a fascial tube surrounding the common and internal carotid arteries and internal jugular vein. Lying within it posteriorly is the vagus nerve. The sheath is in close connection with the prevertebral fascia, with the sympathetic chain intervening. The surface markings are a thick band some 1.5–2 cm wide from the sternoclavicular joint to the tragus. The division of the common carotid lies 1 cm

below and behind the greater cornu of the hyoid at C3–4 vertebral level.
[A:504; E:623; G:934, 937]

151 The internal carotid artery has no branches in the neck, its first branch being the ophthalmic artery. The external carotid artery has numerous large cervical branches to the thyroid, tongue, pharynx, ear, occiput and face.
[I:424; J:170, 172]

152 The vagus nerve, with its many branches to larynx and pharynx, is an immediate posterior relation of the carotid artery, as is the sympathetic chain which lies just outside the carotid sheath on the prevertebral fascia. Both of these nerves may be damaged if the needle penetrates too deeply.
[D:281; F:518; G:936]

H Information answers

153 The vestibule of the mouth is that part which lies external to the gums and teeth. Anterior to it the lips are situated. Laterally is the cheek containing the buccinator. Superiorly and inferiorly the vestibule is limited by the reflection of the mucous membrane of the lips and cheek onto the gums.
[A:1205; C:828; F:566]

154 The tongue is divided into an anterior two-thirds and a posterior one-third by the V-shaped sulcus terminalis. As regards general sensation, the anterior two-thirds is supplied by the lingual nerve (a branch of the mandibular division of the trigeminal); the posterior third is supplied by the glossopharyngeal nerve.
[A:1237; B:716; E:742; G:783]

155 Taste fibres from the anterior two-thirds of the tongue travel in the lingual nerve to the infratemporal fossa. Here they leave it in the chorda tympani to join the facial nerve in the petrous temporal bone. Taste fibres from the posterior third run in the lingual branch of the glossopharyngeal nerve. This nerve also supplies the circumvallate papillae, which are situated immediately anterior to the sulcus termi-

nalis. Taste fibres from the region of the epiglottis and valleculae run in the internal laryngeal branch of the vagus nerve.
[A:1085; E:670, 734; G:781]

156   The muscles of the tongue are divided into two groups: intrinsic and extrinsic. The intrinsic muscles are confined to the tongue itself, are not attached to any bone and serve to alter the shape of the organ. They are arranged in longitudinal, vertical and transverse bundles. The extrinsic muscles are attached to the surrounding skeleton and serve to move the tongue as a whole. They are the genioglossus, hyoglossus, styloglossus and palatoglossus. The genioglossi run from the genial tubercles, on the internal aspect of the mandible, to the tongue. They protrude the tongue. The hyoglossus runs from the upper border of the hyoid, as a quadrilateral sheet, to the tongue. If the hyoid is fixed, contraction of this muscle depresses the tongue. The styloglossus runs from the tip of the styloid process to the tongue, pulling the tongue backwards and upwards upon contraction. The palatoglossus runs from the aponeurosis of the soft palate, down the lateral pharyngeal wall to the tongue. Together they act as a sphincter, closing the oropharyngeal orifice. All the muscles of the tongue (intrinsic and extrinsic) are supplied by the hypoglossal nerve except for palatoglossus, which is supplied by the pharyngeal plexus.
[A:1239; C:844; G:785]

157   The thyroid gland develops as a diverticulum of the floor of the embryological pharynx. The developing tongue overgrows this diverticulum and hence it appears that the diverticulum arises from the tongue. It is therefore called the thyroglossal duct. As the thyroid develops it descends, and the thyroglossal duct atrophies. In the normal individual all that remains is a small pit on the apex of the 'V' of the sulcus terminalis. This is the foramen caecum. Sometimes, however, the thyroid fails to descend and remains in the region of the foramen caecum. This is called a lingual thyroid. Sometimes the thyroglossal duct fails to atrophy completely. Cysts may form in those parts remaining.
[A:169; C:773; D:288]

158 The chorda tympani is a branch of the facial nerve. It leaves the facial nerve in the petrous temporal bone, crosses the tympanic cavity and leaves the skull via the petrotympanic fissure, to enter the infratemporal fossa. In the infratemporal fossa it joins the lingual nerve. The chorda tympani contains two kinds of fibres: taste fibres and preganglionic parasympathetic secretomotor fibres. The taste fibres originate from the anterior two-thirds of the tongue. Their cell bodies are situated in the geniculate ganglion of the facial nerve. The preganglionic parasympathetic fibres are destined for the submandibular ganglion. Here they synapse and are distributed to the sublingual and submandibular salivary glands.
[A:1014; B:620; C:886; H:59]

159 The deciduous teeth do not start to erupt until the sixth month. Therefore a baby of 4 months would have no visible teeth at all. The central deciduous incisors erupt at about 6 months, the lateral incisors at 9 months. The first deciduous molars arrive at 12 months and the canines at 18 months. A child of 20 months would be expected, therefore, to possess all the deciduous incisors and canines and the first molars (the second deciduous molars do not usually erupt until 24 months of age). By the age of 12 years all the deciduous teeth have been replaced by the permanent dentition. Furthermore, all the permanent teeth have erupted by this age, except the third molars (wisdom teeth), which may not arrive until the thirtieth year. Thus a child of 12 years would have—in each half jaw—two incisors, one canine, two premolars and two molars. All of these teeth would be permanent.
[A:1233; F:571; G:797; H:20]

160 All three of the major salivary glands (parotid, submandibular and sublingual) are in direct contact with the mandible. The parotid gland overlies the posterior border of the ramus of the mandible and its adjacent medial and lateral surfaces. The superficial part of the submandibular gland lies in immediate relationship to the submandibular fossa of the mandible. This is situated on the medial aspect of the body, below the mylohyoid line. The sublingual gland

lies in the sublingual fossa on the inner and posterior aspect of the mandible above the mylohyoid line. The following nerves are directly related to the mandible. They are all branches of the mandibular nerve: the lingual nerve, the nerve to mylohyoid, the inferior alveolar nerve and the auriculotemporal nerve. The lingual nerve runs in a groove on the mandible for a short distance, related to the third molar tooth above. The inferior alveolar nerve enters the mandibular foramen and supplies the mandible, teeth and gums. It emerges at the mental foramen as the mental nerve. The nerve to mylohyoid, a branch of the inferior alveolar, runs on the medial aspect of the body of the mandible immediately below the mylohyoid line. It supplies the muscle from its superficial aspect. The auriculotemporal nerve runs posteriorly round the neck of the mandible to reach the temporal region.
[A:281, 1008; B:577; H:23]

161 The submandibular gland consists of two parts: a larger superficial part and a smaller deep part. The two parts are continuous around the free posterior border of mylohyoid, and hence the gland looks like a letter 'C' when removed. The submandibular duct leaves the gland at the anterior extremity of the deep part and passes anteriorly along the floor of the mouth lateral to the tongue, to open into the mouth at the summit of a papilla, situated immediately lateral to the frenulum of the tongue.
[A:1211; E:681; H:38]

162 Preganglionic parasympathetic fibres from the superior salivary nucleus leave the brain in the nervus intermedius in the groove between the pons and the medulla oblongata. The nervus intermedius runs into the internal auditory meatus with nerves VII and VIII and fuses with the facial nerve (VII). Within the petrous temporal bone the parasympathetic fibres destined for the submandibular gland leave the facial nerve in the chorda tympani. The chorda tympani crosses the tympanic membrane and leaves the skull at the petrotympanic fissure, to enter the infratemporal fossa. Here the chorda tympani joins the lingual nerve. Passing in the lingual nerve the parasympathetic fibres reach

the submandibular ganglion, which lies under the lingual nerve, superficial to hyoglossus. In the ganglion the fibres synapse. The postganglionic fibres pass to the submandibular and sublingual glands either directly or in branches of the lingual nerve.
[A:1015; B:676; G:87]

163 In the submandibular region, on the hyoglossus muscle, the submandibular duct (Wharton) passes forwards to enter the mouth. The lingual nerve crosses it from superior to inferior on its lateral aspect. It then immediately winds underneath the duct and crosses it from inferior to superior on its medial aspect, to reach the tongue. This 'double-crossing' of Wharton's duct by the lingual nerve is remembered by most students, as it is immortalised in a ribald rhyming mnemonic.
[A:1211; G:788; H:44]

H Applied answers

164 A midline congenital tumour in the region of the foramen caecum, though rare, is quite likely to be a lingual thyroid remnant. This may turn out to be the only thyroid tissue the child possesses. The histology will consist of colloid-filled thyroid follicles whose walls are made up of a single layer of cuboid epithelium.
[A:169; D:285]

165 The genioglossus muscles originate from the genial tubercle or mental spine of the mandible and spread out like a fan backwards into the bulk of the tongue. In the unconscious patient the tongue falls back, blocking the airway, and the simplest way to stop this is to push the angle of the jaw forwards. In doing so, the genioglossi are pulled anteriorly and the bulk of the tongue is removed from the oropharynx.
[G:788; H:45]

166 Within the distribution of the trigeminal nerve, referred pain from one region to another is quite a common symptom. In this case, the lingual nerve to the tongue is being stimulated

by the mouth lesion but the pain is being felt through the auriculotemporal nerve to the ear.
[E:670; G:781]

167 The anterior two-thirds of the tongue is drained by lymphatics to its ipsilateral submental and submandibular nodes, whereas the posterior third of the tongue has many lymphatic anastomoses across the midline which drain to the upper deep cervical nodes. A posterior tumour is therefore more likely to spread to contralateral nodes. The rationale to the lymphatic drainage is due to a partial midline septum in the anterior two-thirds.
[D:293; E:640; G:913]

168 When asked to put out the tongue, a right hypoglossal palsy would be seen as an atrophy of the right side accompanied by deviation of the tongue towards the affected side.
[C:828; G:788]

169 In removing the lower wisdom teeth it is quite easy to traumatise the lingual nerve as it runs on the mylohyoid muscle just medial to the roots of the lower wisdom teeth. Damage to this nerve affects not only the sensory supply from the anterior two-thirds of the tongue but also all the fibres carried by the chorda tympani. Proximal to the molar teeth, deep in the infratemporal fossa, the chorda tympani joins the lingual nerve carrying the special sensory (taste) fibres from the anterior part of the tongue as well as the preganglionic parasympathetic secretomotor fibres to the submandibular and sublingual glands. Damage to these fibres will alter the normal salivary secretions, which patients may notice as a funny metallic taste. This taste is probably due to an imbalance of ions due to changed salivary concentrations.
[E:669; G:781; H:38]

170 The taste fibres in the chorda tympani are the peripheral processes of the geniculate ganglion cells and any tumour within the middle ear may affect either the chorda tympani or the ganglion itself. The geniculate ganglion lies above the promontory on the medial wall of the middle ear whilst the chorda tympani lies between the

malleus and incus on the medial side of the tympanic membrane.
[E:736; G:7159; H:59]

171 In general, girls' teeth erupt slightly earlier than boys' and the lower jaw before the upper, but by the age of 22 the majority of students would have their third molar or wisdom teeth. If the third molars did not require removal due to impaction, a full set of adult teeth is 32 teeth. However, some people's wisdom teeth do not erupt until 24 years or beyond. The normal range for the appearance of these four teeth is 16–30 years.
[C:830; G:7103]

172 The mental nerve which supplies the lower lip is a branch of the inferior alveolar nerve which lies inside the mandible supplying the teeth. Any jaw fracture might therefore cause loss of sensation over the chin and lower lip.
[G:717]

173 The lower lip musculature is supplied by the cervical and mandibular branches of the facial nerve. In operating on a submandibular growth it may be impossible to avoid cutting through either or both of these nerves, leaving the patient with a drooped lip.
[D:395; G:767; H:36]

174 On putting the tip of the tongue up to the roof of the mouth, a prominent midline fold of mucous membrane—the frenulum—can be seen. On either side of the frenulum are the sublingual papillae, on the surface of which can be found the opening of the submandibular duct (Wharton). Lying lateral to the papillae are the sublingual folds, beneath which lie the sublingual glands whose numerous ducts open along the crest of the folds. A few drops of lemon juice on the tongue may produce a jet of saliva from the submandibular duct orifices.
[B:719; E:743; G:788]

I Information answers

175 The floor of the posterior triangle is formed by muscles, covered by the prevertebral layer of

deep cervical fascia. From superior to inferior, these muscles are semispinalis capitis, splenius capitis, levator scapulae and the three scalenes (medius, posterior and anterior).
[A:505; F:464; H:35]

176 The posterior triangle of the neck is situated with its apex superiorly and its base inferiorly. It is bounded inferiorly by the middle third of the clavicle, anteriorly by the posterior border of the sternomastoid and posteriorly by the anterior border of trapezius. Its roof is the investing layer of the deep cervical fascia, covered in turn by superficial fascia, containing the platysma and skin.
[A:505, 632; H:33]

177 The deep cervical chain of nodes which drain the structures of the head and neck are situated under cover of the sternomastoid muscle along the internal jugular vein. Clinically, they are difficult to feel unless the sternomastoid is relaxed.
[A:729; H:38]

178 The sensory branches of the cervical plexus are the lesser occipital nerve, the greater auricular nerve, the transverse cervical nerve and the supraclavicular nerves. They all appear in the posterior triangle behind the posterior border of the sternomastoid. The lesser occipital nerve (C2) hooks round the anterior aspect of the accessory nerve in the posterior triangle. It ascends up the posterior border of the sternomastoid to supply skin behind the ear and around the mastoid process. The greater auricular nerve (C2, 3) appears in the posterior triangle at the posterior border of the sternomastoid. It passes anterosuperiorly onto the muscle and ascends in company with the external jugular vein. It supplies skin over the angle of the mandible and the parotid region. The transverse cervical nerve (C2, 3) appears behind the posterior border of the sternomastoid and passes anteriorly over the muscle to supply the skin of the front of the neck. The supraclavicular nerves (C3, 4) are usually three in number —lateral, intermediate and medial. They pass posteroinferiorly across the clavicle to supply

the skin of the upper chest and deltoid region.
They may actually pierce the clavicle.
[A:1034; G:94; H:36]

179   C1 has no cutaneous branch and therefore normally has no dermatome.
[A:1062; G:533]

I Applied answers

180   The posterior triangle of the neck is bounded by
the clavicle, sternomastoid and trapezius muscles. Its superior half contains few structures of
significance except for the spinal part of the
accessory nerve and sensory branches of the
cervical plexus. The inferior portion, however,
contains not only the trunks of the brachial
plexus, lying deep to omohyoid muscle, but
also the subclavian vein and artery. Both of
these vessels have numerous branches in the
posterior triangle, the suprascapular and transverse cervical being two of the more vulnerable
vessels.
[E:622; G:94; H:33]

181   The spinal part of the accessory nerve supplies
the sternomastoid and trapezius muscles. It
traverses the posterior triangle lying rather
superficially in the cervical investing fascia and
is quite easily damaged if an incision is made
transversely across the triangle. Damage to the
trapezius innervation makes elevation movements of the shoulder in abduction very difficult.
[E:626; G:95, 732; H:69]

182   Leprosy (Hansen's disease) is a systemic infection with a predeliction for nerves, causing loss
of sensation, depigmentation and thickening of
peripheral nerves. These swollen nerves are felt
as lumps or cords under the skin. An often
visible abnormality is swelling of the greater
auricular nerve (C2, 3) which supplies the angle
of the jaw, mastoid region, side of the neck and
both surfaces of the ear.
[E:626; G:94; H:35]

183   There are numerous inconstant venous channels between the brain and scalp but there are

also at least six paired emissary veins, the most constant being those found in the parietal, mastoid and condylar regions. There is also often a large unpaired occipital emissary vein near the external occipital protuberance. There are therefore numerous venous connections of the occipital region with the intracranial venous sinuses, providing an easy path for the spread of infection.
[E:652; F:480; G:720]

184 Deep in the floor of the suboccipital triangle lies an important source of blood supply to the brain—the vertebral artery. Bounded by the small rotator muscles of the neck and lying on the posterior arch of the atlas, the vertebral artery ascends through the foramen transversarium of C1, turns medially prior to penetrating the posterior atlanto-occipital membrane and then ascends through the foramen magnum.
[A:514; G:536]

J   Information answers

185 The parietal pleura rises up into the neck to the level of the neck of the first rib. In this area it is termed the cervical pleura. Its surface marking is a curved line joining the sternoclavicular joint to the lateral extremity of the medial third of the clavicle. This line should extend 2.5 cm above the clavicle at its maximum convexity. The cervical pleura is covered by the suprapleural membrane (Sibson's fascia), which is attached to the inner margin of the first rib and separates the root of the neck from the thorax. The subclavian vessels arch over this membrane.
[A:1192; E:70; G:124]

186 The branches of the subclavian artery are: the vertebral artery, internal thoracic artery, thyrocervical trunk, costocervical trunk and dorsal scapular artery. With the exception of the dorsal scapular branch, on both sides, and the costocervical branch, on the right, all the branches arise from the first part of the artery—i.e. medial to scalenus anterior. The vertebral artery enters the foramina transversarium of C6 and ascends through successive foramina transversaria. It winds posterior to the lateral mass of

the atlas and enters the foramen magnum. It supplies the posterior parts of the brain. The internal thoracic artery descends behind the costal cartilages of the ribs, supplying the intercostal spaces and surrounding structures. The thyrocervical trunk divides into inferior thyroid, suprascapular and superficial cervical arteries. The costocervical trunk divides into deep cervical and superior intercostal arteries. The dorsal scapular artery supplies a small amount of blood to the anastomosis around the scapula. [A:639; E:392; G:938]

187 The vertebral artery arises from the first part of the subclavian artery. It runs upwards between the longus cervicis and scalene muscles, passes anterior to the transverse process of C7 and enters the foramen transversarium of C6. It ascends in successive foramina transversaria until the atlas is reached. The atlas has no foramen transversarium so the artery winds behind its lateral mass, in the suboccipital triangle, then turns medially and pierces the dura to lie in the vertebral canal. It then passes upwards and enters the skull through the foramen magnum. In the skull it runs upwards, forwards and medially between the medulla and clivus. At the upper border of the medulla it fuses with its fellow to form the basilar artery. By convention, the vertebral artery is divided into four parts. The first part extends from the subclavian artery to the transverse process of C6. The second part is that where the artery lies in the foramina transversaria. The third part is in the suboccipital triangle, and the fourth part is the intracranial portion. [A:641; E:638; G:539, 712]

188 The recurrent laryngeal nerves arise from the vagus nerves but at different levels on the two sides. The right recurrent laryngeal nerve arises from the right vagus as it crosses anterior to the first part of the subclavian artery. It hooks round under the right subclavian artery and ascends between the trachea and oesophagus to the larynx. The left recurrent laryngeal nerve arises from the left vagus as the latter crosses anterior to the aortic arch. It loops beneath the ligamentum arteriosum and ascends between the trachea and oesophagus to the larynx.

Developmentally, the recurrent laryngeal nerves are the nerves of the sixth pharyngeal pouches. They are therefore associated with the sixth pharyngeal arch arteries. As the neck enlarges and the heart descends, these vessels are pulled inferiorly and the nerves with them so the nerves now take a recurrent course downwards, round the vessel and upwards again. On the left side, the sixth arch artery becomes the ductus arteriosus. The left recurrent laryngeal nerve therefore runs round this vessel which, in adult life, is obliterated to a fibrous cord, the ligamentum arteriosum. On the right, the sixth and fifth arch arteries disappear. The right recurrent laryngeal nerve therefore loops round the next most superior vessel, which is the right fourth arch artery. This vessel develops into the proximal portion of the right subclavian artery, which the right recurrent laryngeal nerve is seen to run round.
[A:160; D:39; F:440]

189 The thoracic duct is a major lymphatic vessel recognised by its beaded appearance due to the presence of numerous valves. It commences at the upper border of the cisterna chyli, which is situated on the posterior abdominal wall at L1 on the right of the aorta. The thoracic duct ascends through the aortic hiatus of the diaphragm into the thorax. At the level of T4 it crosses to the left-hand side of the vertebral column, passing behind all the longitudinally running thoracic structures as it does so, and comes eventually to lie on the left of the oesophagus. In this position it continues to ascend into the neck. At the level of C7 it arches laterally, and then turns downwards, passing anterior to all the major arterial vessels of the neck, to end by draining into the confluence of the internal jugular and subclavian veins.
[A:727; G:940; H:191]

190 The cervical sympathetic trunk possesses three ganglia, termed superior cervical, middle cervical and inferior cervical. The superior cervical ganglion is derived from cord segments C1–4, the middle from C5–6 and the inferior from C7–8. The inferior ganglion is frequently fused with the upper thoracic ganglion to form the stellate ganglion. The superior ganglion is

situated at the level of the hyoid bone, the
inferior around the neck of the first rib. The
efferent branches are of three kinds: grey rami
communicantes, direct branches and vascular
branches. Each cervical spinal nerve receives a
grey ramus communicans from its respective
ganglion. The superior cervical ganglion sends
direct branches to the first four cranial nerves,
the pharynx and the cardiac plexus. It also
sends vascular branches with the external carotid arteries and their branches. A further
branch, the internal carotid nerve, accompanies
the internal carotid artery through the carotid
canal. The middle cervical ganglion sends a
direct branch to the cardiac plexus and a vascular branch to the thyroid gland along the inferior thyroid artery. The inferior ganglion also
sends a direct branch to the cardiac plexus and
vascular branches to the subclavian and vertebral arteries. The trunk itself divides on either
side of the subclavian artery to form the ansa
subclavia.
[A:1070; D:328; G:946]

191   The scalenus anterior is a cervical muscle of the
prevertebral group. This means that it will lie
posterior to any viscera or vessels in the neck. It
is covered anteriorly by the prevertebral fascia.
Between the muscle and the fascia is situated
the phrenic nerve as it descends towards the
thorax. Anterior to this musculoskeletal plane,
there is in the neck an arterial plane in which
the transverse cervical artery is situated. The
thoracic duct is anterior to this arterial plane.
Thus the order of structures from posterior to
anterior is: scalenus anterior, phrenic nerve,
transverse cervical artery and thoracic duct.
[A:1036; E:638]

192   The trunks of the brachial plexus and subclavian artery and vein all cross the superior surface of the first rib to enter the arm. The lower
trunk of the brachial plexus is derived from
roots C8 and T1, which arise on either side of
the first rib. This means that the lower trunk is
actually in contact with the rib's upper surface.
The subclavian vessels also are in contact with
the superior surface as they arch over the rib
and descend into the arm. Of these structures,
the subclavian vein is the most anterior. The

subclavian artery is posterior to the vein but separated from it by the insertion of scalenus anterior at the scalene tubercle. The nerves are posterior to these vessels. Thus the lower trunk of the brachial plexus lies posterior to the artery. In summary, the order of structures from anterior to posterior is: subclavian vein, subclavian artery and lower trunk of brachial plexus.
[A:252, 689; E:638]

193 The first rib is the shortest of all the ribs and has the most pronounced curve. It is flattened superoinferiorly and hence possesses medial and lateral edges. Normal ribs are flattened mediolaterally and have superior and inferior edges. The first rib has a scalene tubercle on its medial border (edge) for the insertion of scalenus anterior. This muscle separates the subclavian artery posteriorly from the subclavian vein anteriorly at this point. Both the above vessels can be seen to groove the upper surface of the first rib, a feature possessed by no other rib. The head of the first rib is small and round. It articulates with one vertebral body only (that of T1), and hence bears only one articular facet.
[A:252; G:939; H:151]

J Applied answers

194 Insertion of a needle into the angle formed by the confluence of the internal jugular and subclavian veins might well encounter the terminal portion of the thoracic duct. The brachiocephalic route for a central venous catheterisation on the left-hand side has been known to cause a chylothorax.
[B:331; E:649; G:938, 940; J:222]

195 The muscles involved in shoulder abduction are primarily the deltoid with assistance from supraspinatus. The nerve supply to the deltoid is the axillary nerve from the posterior cord of the brachial plexus which lies around the neck of the humerus. The supraspinatus muscle, however, is innervated by the suprascapular nerve (C5, 6) which is derived directly from the upper trunk. Without the supraspinatus the initial component of abduction is weakened, and the more one tries to abduct the arm, the

more one shrugs the shoulder. This is because the supraspinatus holds the humeral head into the glenoid fossa and stops it sliding in abduction.
[F:158; G:639; H:112]

196 The immediate posterior relationship of the great veins of the neck is the cupola of the pleura and apex of the lung. Posteriorly, this is the level of the first rib. However, as the ribs slope downwards, the pleura extends above the first rib anteriorly. Just posterior to the sterno-mastoid muscle the pleural dome lies some 2–3 cm above the medial third of the clavicle. In this region the cupola of the pleura is strengthened by a fascial thickening called the suprapleural membrane (Sibson's fascia). Any catheterisation that misses the veins and continues posteriorly may produce a pneumothorax.
[B:274; E:638; G:938; H:190]

197 The inferior cervical and first thoracic sympathetic ganglia are often amalgamated to form the cervicothoracic or stellate ganglion just posterior to the origin of the vertebral artery. A cervical or upper thoracic sympathectomy will cut off the sympathetic innervation to the whole of the head and neck of the same side. This leaves the patient with a hot, dry, flushed face with no capacity to sweat, ptosis of the eyelid, constriction of the pupil and retraction of the eye (enophthalmos)—Horner's syndrome. For this reason, when performing thoracic sympathectomies for vascular problems in the upper limb, it is very wise to try to avoid the stellate ganglion!
[A:1073; G:946; H:41]

198 Occasionally, the seventh cervical vertebra has a fully developed rib which may articulate with the manubrium sterni. More commonly, however, is a remnant of the cartilaginous rib found *in utero*. The incidence has been estimated at about 0.5 per cent but it is more important to realise that this condition is one of the factors involved in thoracic inlet syndromes. These may present as vascular insufficiency in the hand or tingling in the fingers due to pressure in the neck on the lower trunk of the brachial plexus.
[C:496; E:63; G:17]

K Information answers

199 The outer aspect of the pinna is supplied with
nerves from two sources. The anterosuperior
half is supplied by the auriculotemporal nerve,
a branch of the trigeminal (V). The posteroinferior half is supplied by the greater auricular
nerve (C2, 3) from the cervical plexus. The back
of the pinna is supplied mostly by the lesser
occipital nerve (C2). The greater auricular supplies the inferior part adjacent to the lobule. The
vagus supplies a small strip of skin posteriorly
at the root of the pinna.

For the purpose of description of its nerve
supply, the tympanic membrane is divided into
anterior and posterior halves. The anterior half
is supplied by the auriculotemporal nerve (V).
The posterior half is supplied by the vagus (X).
[A:1136, 1145; E:621, 730; H:58]

200 The tympanic membrane is connected to the
handle of the malleus. The head of the malleus
articulates with the body of the incus. The incus
in turn articulates via its long process with the
head of the stapes. The footplate of the stapes
rests in the fenestra ovalis. The bones of the
tympanic cavity are held in place by ligaments:
one runs from the short process of the incus to
the posterior wall, another from the anterior
process of the malleus to the anterior wall of the
cavity. The ossicles act like a gearbox, converting vibrations of the tympanic membrane into
in-and-out piston-like movements where the
stapes is inserted into the fenestra ovalis (vestibuli).
[A:1143; E:734; G:7152; H:58]

201 The mastoid antrum lies in front of the sigmoid
venous sinus and the cerebellum. Infection in
the region of the mastoid may spread to involve
these structures.
[A:1141; G:7157; H:59]

202 The most obvious feature of the medial wall of
the middle ear is a convex bulge termed the
promontory. This is caused by the underlying
first turn of the cochlea. The fenestra ovalis
(fenestra vestibuli) lies superoposterior to the
promontory. It is for articulation with the footplate of the stapes. Posteroinferior to the promontory lies the fenestra rotunda (fenestra

cochleae) covered by its membrane. A ridge may be seen running posteriorly from the region above the promontory to the posterior wall of the tympanic cavity. The ridge is caused by the underlying facial nerve (that part distal to the geniculate ganglion). A ridge of bone is seen running to the area above the promontory from the anterior wall of the middle ear. This ridge of bone supports the tensor tympani muscle. It ends in a pulley (processus cochleariformis) for the tendon to run round in order to pass laterally to the handle of the malleus.
[A:1140; E:736; G:7150; H:59]

203 The facial nerve enters the petrous temporal bone via the internal acoustic meatus in company with the vestibulocochlear nerve. At the bottom of the meatus it enters a tunnel, the facial canal. The nerve runs laterally above the vestibule of the inner ear until it reaches the medial wall of the tympanic cavity above the promontory. Here it bends 90° and runs posteriorly towards the posterior wall of the tympanic cavity. A swelling is associated with this abrupt bend—the geniculate ganglion. At the posterior wall it bends again through 90°, this time to turn inferiorly, and running downwards is situated in the medial wall of the aditus. It continues inferiorly along the posterior tympanic wall and leaves the skull at the stylomastoid foramen.
[A:1011; E:736; G:7159; H:60]

204 The branches of the facial nerve in the petrous temporal bone are the greater petrosal nerve, the nerve to stapedius and the chorda tympani.

The greater petrosal nerve contains preganglionic parasympathetic fibres destined for the sphenopalatine ganglion. From here, postganglionic fibres are distributed to the lacrimal gland and glands of the nose.

The nerve to stapedius is motor to the stapedius muscle, which runs from the pyramid of the posterior tympanic wall to the neck of the stapes. Its contraction 'damps down' movements of the stapes and prevents damage to the inner ear should it be bombarded with loud noises.

The chorda tympani contains two sets of fibres. One set comprises the taste fibres from the anterior two-thirds of the tongue. The other

set contains preganglionic parasympathetic fibres destined for the submandibular ganglion where they synapse and are distributed to the sublingual and submandibular salivary glands.
[A:1012; E:736; G:7163; H:49]

205 The membranous labyrinth is a freely communicating collection of sacs and ducts which lie within the cavity of the bony labyrinth and are separated from them by perilymph. The membranous labyrinth itself contains endolymph.

From anterior to posterior, it consists of the duct of the cochlea, the saccule and utricle and the semicircular ducts. The duct of the cochlea is situated within the bony cochlea. It contains the basilar membrane which has special hair cells for the appreciation of sound—the organ of Corti. The semicircular ducts lie within the bony semicircular canals. The utricle and saccule are the two central chambers of the membranous labyrinth. They contain the sense organs for the appreciation of the direction of gravity. Their terminations with the utricle contain swellings termed ampullae. It is here that special sense organs are situated to detect acceleration occurring in each of the planes represented by the semicircular canals.

The saccus endolymphaticus is a blind-ended diverticulum of the central portion of the membranous labyrinth.
[A:1149; E:736; G:7169]

206 There are three semicircular canals in each inner ear: superior, posterior and lateral. The lateral canal is set in the horizontal plane, its convexity directed laterally. The superior canal is situated vertically, in the axis of the petrous temporal bone which is anteromedial to posterolateral. The posterior canal is also set vertically but at 90° to the petrous temporal axis; therefore, it runs anterolateral to posteromedial. Thus the posterior canal of one ear is set in the same plane as the superior canal of the opposite ear and vice versa.
[A:1146, 1149; G:7162; H:59; J:30]

207 The cochlea consists of a central modiolus around which a hollow cone is wrapped two and a half times. The cochlear nerve ascends in the modiolus and is distributed to each success-

ive turn of the modiolus. A ridge projects into the cavity of the cochlea (the spinal lamina), causing the cavity to be kidney shaped. The duct of the cochlea is triangular shaped in cross-section. Its apex is attached to the spinal lamina and its base to the middle third of the outer surface of the bony cochlea. It is filled with endolymph. Its inferior margin is the basilar membrane which supports the organ of Corti. Above and below the duct of the cochlea are two triangular spaces—the scala vestibuli and scala tympani, respectively. They are filled with perilymph and are in communication over the apex of the cochlear duct. The scala vestibuli ends in the fenestra ovale on which the stapes impinges. The scala tympani ends in the secondary tympanic membrane over the fenestra rotunda.

[A:1147, 1153; F:596; G:7168; H:60]

K Applied answers

208 The external ear consists of the auricle and external auditory meatus. The auricle is composed of fibrocartilage covered closely by skin. The lobule, or ear lobe, is the only part of the auricle with intervening connective tissue, and is often stretched to accommodate ear rings, plugs or other traditional finery. The most obvious features of the auricle are the outer rounded lip—the helix—surrounding the fossae which in turn give way to the inner lip or antihelix. Protecting the entrance of the external auditory meatus is a prominent projection, the tragus. The auricular cartilage is continuous with the cartilaginous lateral third of the canal itself. One should note that, at birth, the external auditory meatus is entirely cartilaginous except for the roof. In the adult, however, the medial two-thirds is part of the temporal bone. The entire canal is lined by skin which is closely applied to the bony canal but is separated from the cartilaginous portion by subcutaneous tissue containing numerous ceruminous glands which produce wax.

[E:731; G:7143; H:58]

209 The tympanic membrane is situated at the medial end of the external auditory meatus, sepa-

rating it from the ossicles of the middle ear. It is a roundish structure facing downwards and forwards, but the effect of parallax makes it appear oval when seen through the otoscope. The normal membrane is glistening and semi-opaque, and the handle of malleus can be seen attached to its deep surface. Occasionally, posteriorly, the incus shadow can be visualised. From the lateral process of the malleus the anterior and posterior malleolar folds form the margin of a lax membrane, the pars flaccida. The remaining membrane is taut and concave where the handle of the malleus pulls it inwards. This area is called the pars tensa and the point of maximum concavity the umbo. On examination, a reflected 'cone of light' from the otoscope is seen in the anteroinferior part of the membrane.
[D:407; E:731; G:7151; H:58]

210 The external auditory meatus is S-shaped; the first part passes forwards and upwards, the second is slightly backwards and the longest third part runs forwards and slightly downwards. To straighten out this canal in the adult, gentle traction is applied in an upwards and backwards direction. In the infant, pulling downwards and backwards is more rewarding.
[C:882; F:591; G:7144]

211 The nerve supply of the canal and tympanic membrane, especially in the posterior and inferior portions, is via the tiny auricular branch of the vagus nerve. This nerve may also carry glossopharyngeal and facial nerve fibres, and some people who are particularly sensitive to stimulation of these nerves may well develop an ear-cough reflex or occasional vomiting which may be associated with the vagal and glossopharyngeal innervation. Sometimes even a persistent lump of wax against the tympanic membrane may be the cause of an unexplained cough.
[B:615; E:736; G:7159]

212 A Ramsay Hunt syndrome is a herpes zoster infection of the geniculate ganglion, also involving cranial nerves IX and X, which causes vesicles to appear in the distribution of the auricular branch of the vagus nerve. This there-

fore suggests that there are general **sensory** fibres of the facial nerve carried with the vagus branches to the auricle and external auditory meatus. In this syndrome one sometimes also finds vesicles on the palate and pharynx.
[F:597; G:87, 7163; H:58]

213 Hyperacusis is seen when the stapedius muscle of the middle ear is not functioning properly and cannot therefore damp down the stapes vibrations. An unusual taste in the mouth may have many causes though damage to the chorda tympani with abnormal salivary secretions is a possible cause. Facial weakness at once makes one think of a VIIth cranial nerve lesion, which could also explain the first two symptoms if the lesion is proximal to the middle ear from where the nerve to stapedius and the chorda tympani branch. Vertigo has various causes—both labyrinthine and cerebral—but taken together with the deafness, a likely diagnosis would be a lesion affecting both the VIIth and VIIIth cranial nerves. Clinically, these occur quite often as a tumour in the cerebellopontine angle arising from the sheath of the vestibular portion of the VIIIth nerve (acoustic neuroma). Other cranial nerves may also be involved, especially the VIth nerve presenting as a lateral rectus palsy.
[E:736; G:731; H:67]

214 In children an untreated otitis media may spread to the mastoid air cells. From here the infection may well break through the superior wall of the mastoid and into the cranial cavity, affecting the meninges and temporal lobe, and causing meningitis or a temporal lobe abscess. If the posterior wall of the mastoid antrum is invaded, the sigmoid dural venous sinus may be infected, causing a thrombosis with all its very serious consequences. Meningitis, cerebral abscess or venous sinus thrombosis could all cause the symptoms and signs described.
[E:736; F:593; G:7161]

215 Commercially it is good for business but, anatomically, the reason is that swallowing opens up the auditory tube (Eustachian, pharyngotympanic). The auditory tube allows equalisation of pressure from the middle ear to the

outside world. When taking off, and particularly when descending in an aircraft, the pressure changes are quite noticeable, and unless the tube is opened the increased air pressure inside the middle ear may cause quite considerable pain. This also explains why flying with a cold can be uncomfortable, as the mucous secretions may block the auditory tube, causing increased pressure within the middle ear. The exact mechanism of opening the tube is debated, but during swallowing the pharyngeal walls are raised and one of the contributing muscles is salpingopharyngeus which originates from the pharyngeal end of the cartilaginous tube.

[F:591; G:7157; H:47]

UPPER LIMB

A Information answers

216 The axillary sheath is a fibrous sheath which encloses the first part of the axillary artery and the adjacent parts of the axillary vein and brachial plexus. It is a prolongation of the prevertebral layer of the deep cervical fascia.
[A:648; G:618]

217 The axilla is the shape of a triangular pyramid with its top cut off. The apex of the axilla is situated superiorly and is in continuity with the neck. Its boundaries are: medially the first rib, anteriorly the clavicle and posteriorly the superior border of the scapula. The axillary blood vessels and brachial plexus enter the upper limb through this triangular space. The walls of the axilla are posterior, anterior and medial. The posterior wall consists of the scapula, covered by the subscapularis above and the latissimus dorsi and teres major below. The anterior wall is formed by the pectoralis major and minor, and clavipectoral fascia where the latter muscle is absent. The medial wall consists of the upper four ribs and intercostal spaces, filled by the intercostal muscles, and the upper half of the serratus anterior muscle. The base is formed by skin and a thick layer of fascia (the axillary fascia) sealing the walls. The axilla contains the axillary vessels, the lower portion of the bra-

chial plexus and its branches, lymph nodes and fat.
[A:647; E:374; G:622; H:118]

218   The medial cord of the brachial plexus is situated medial to the second part of the axillary artery. Its branches are the medial pectoral nerve and the medial cutaneous nerves of the arm and the forearm. It terminates by dividing into two—the ulnar nerve and the medial root of the median nerve. The posterior cord lies posterior to the second part of the axillary artery. Its branches are the upper and lower subscapular nerves and the thoracodorsal nerve (to latissimus dorsi). It ends by dividing into two—the axillary and radial nerves.
[A:1038; G:624; H:118]

219   The brachial plexus is formed from the anterior primary rami of C5–T1. In the neck the trunks are formed, the upper from the union of C5 and C6 roots, the lower from the union of C8 and T1, and the middle by the continuation of C7. Behind the clavicle each trunk divides into two—an anterior and posterior division. All the posterior divisions unite to form the posterior cord. The anterior divisions of the upper and middle trunks join to form the lateral cord, and the anterior division of the lower trunk continues as the medial cord. The cords of the brachial plexus (lateral, posterior and medial) derive their names from their relationship to the second part of the axillary artery around which they are disposed.
[A:1038; D:204; E:382]

220   The area of skin supplied by a single spinal nerve constitutes a dermatome. Dermatome C5 is situated on the lateral aspect of the shoulder and arm, extending as far inferiorly as the elbow joint. The C6 dermatome is situated on the lateral aspect of the forearm. It includes the thumb.
[A:1040; D:205; G:541]

221   The female breast is situated in the superficial fascia of the front and side of the chest. Its usual surface marking is from the second to sixth rib vertically and from the sternum medially to the mid-axillary line laterally. It therefore overlies

pectoralis major, part of serratus anterior and a small portion of the external oblique. The breast is supported by fibrous septa which run from the fascia overlying the gland into its depths— the suspensory ligaments (Astley Cooper).
[A:1364; G:612; H:152]

222   The lymphatic vessels of the breast originate in a subcutaneous subareolar plexus and a deep plexus overlying the muscle bed. From here the lymphatics run with the blood vessels which supply the gland. Thus some 75 per cent of the lymph runs to the axilla (in the same direction as the lateral thoracic artery) and drains to the pectoral (anterior) nodes, and thence to the apical axillary nodes and subclavian trunk. Most of the remainder of the lymph runs with the perforating branches of the internal thoracic artery to the parasternal nodes adjacent to the latter artery and deep to the rib cage. Pathologically, blockage of lymphatics by tumour tissue can cause anastomoses to open up and allow drainage to other areas; for instance, to the opposite breast or the inguinal region.
[A:734; E:368]

A   Applied answers

223   The skin of the upper limb is drained by the lymphatics in a similar manner to the venous drainage. The skin of the fingers is therefore likely to drain via the dorsal digital lymphatics along the forearm to the cubital fossa, where the majority of vessels follow the basilic vein, through the deep fascia and into the lateral groups of axillary nodes.
[E:401; J:218]

224   A cervical rib, in some cases, may cause pressure on the lowest trunk of the brachial plexus or, more commonly, on the T1 nerve root itself. The T1 myotome is to the intrinsic muscles of the hand, and thus wasting of these muscles may occur in cervical rib cases. The dorsal interossei when atrophied cause a noticeable 'guttering' of the fingers.
[G:17; H:141]

225 An Erb's palsy is classically due to an upper trunk lesion, thus affecting C5 and C6 nerve roots. The damaged arm is held in the 'waiter's tip' position with the shoulder adducted, the elbow extended and the hand pronated. This can be explained by damage to the axillary nerve C5, 6 causing an adducted shoulder, as well as damage to the musculocutaneous nerve affecting biceps and brachialis causing loss of elbow flexion and supination.
[D:210; E:472]

226 A 'winged' scapula is seen in some thin women, but following a radical mastectomy one must immediately think of a damaged serratus anterior muscle. The most likely cause is trauma to the long thoracic nerve (Bell) which lies along the medial axillary wall, sending twigs to each of the eight slips of the muscle. It is here that breast surgeons may traumatise it while clearing lymph nodes from the axillary fat.
[E:472; G:628; H:117]

227 If the whole brachial plexus were destroyed, no fibres from C5 to T1 would be capable of sensory appreciation. The bulk of the upper shoulder, however, is supplied by C3 and C4 and these dermatomes are thus unaffected. Remember the distribution of referred pain from the diaphragm.
[G:541; H:108]

228 The axillary nerve arises from the posterior cord of the brachial plexus and divides at the lower border of teres minor into an anterior and posterior branch. The anterior branch, accompanied by the posterior circumflex humeral vessels, winds posteriorly through the quadriquadrangular space and round the surgical neck of the humerus to supply deltoid from its deep surface. This is usually some 6–8 cm inferior to the bony prominence of the acromion. Any injections below and posterior to the midpoint of the acromion will endanger the axillary nerve. Muscular and financial incapacity may result!
[E:408; G:639]

229 Klumpke's paralysis is due to a traction lesion of C8 and T1, giving rise to wasting of intrinsic hand muscles and eventually a claw-hand. Loss

of sensation may also occur along the ulnar side of the hand, forearm and arm.
[D:212; E:472]

230 Tethering is due to shortening of the suspensory ligaments (Cooper) which normally fix the breast tissue to skin and underlying fascia. Tumours within the breast may cause shortening and thus pull the skin inwards, creating a dimple.
[G:612]

231 Peau d'orange is due to cutaneous lymphatic oedema and is a classic sign of advanced carcinoma of the breast. However, anatomically, it is due to a blockage in the normal lymphatic drainage from the breast, mainly to the axillary nodes, and can even be seen in chronic breast abscesses.
[C:177]

232 The whole breast is enlarged, the axillary tail often being noticeable for the first time, and many dilated veins can be seen over the breast skin. The nipple and areola are well pigmented and normally there is a greatly increased number of areolar glands (sebaceous glands of Montgomery). These glands also increase in size, as their function is to lubricate the nipple during lactation.
[H:152]

233 The most likely path for an areolar condition to spread is via the subareolar plexus to the anterior (pectoral) axillary lymph nodes. Often some large lymphatic vessels can be seen to drain from the nipple along the level of the third rib to the axilla. However, lymphatic spread may sometimes involve the parasternal nodes or the opposite breast and even the mediastinal or peritoneal nodes.
[D:170; E:368]

B Information answers

234 The axillary artery commences at the lateral border of the first rib as the continuation of the subclavian artery. It ends at the inferior border of the teres major muscle, continuing as the

brachial artery. It is divided into three parts by the pectoralis minor muscle. The first part is proximal to the muscle, the second part is behind the muscle and the third part distal to it. Conveniently, the first part has one branch, the second part two and the third part three branches. These are the supreme thoracic from the first part, the thoracoacromial and lateral thoracic from the second part, and the anterior and posterior circumflex humeral and subscapular artery from the third part. The subscapular artery is the largest branch. The anastomoses around the scapula bring the subclavian, axillary and upper intercostal arteries into contact. They are necessary to allow adequate perfusion of the upper limb in all positions of the shoulder, when occlusion of the main trunk may occur. The subclavian artery gives two branches to the anastomosis—the suprascapular artery and the deep branch of the transverse cervical. These anastomose on the scapula with the subscapular branch of the axillary artery and with the posterior intercostal arteries over which the scapula lies.
[A:647; E:393]

235 The clavicle can be divided into a medial two-thirds convex anteriorly and a lateral third convex posteriorly. The medial end is rounded for articulation with the sternum, the lateral end flattened for articulation with the acromion. The superior surface of the bone is relatively smooth, but the inferior aspect is roughened by various features. Laterally is a ridge for the attachment of the trapezoid ligament, ending in a tubercle for the conoid ligament. Furthermore, there is a distinct groove for subclavius and a tubercle medially for the costoclavicular ligament. Using these criteria, the side of a clavicle may be easily ascertained.
[A:322; F:153]

236 Two movements are associated with abduction of the arm to 180°—abduction of the glenohumeral joint and rotation of the scapula and entire upper limb. Abduction of the glenohumeral joint is limited to 90°, being initiated by supraspinatus and continued by the middle fibres of deltoid. In order to prevent the head of the humerus being pulled bodily upwards by deltoid during this movement, the teres muscles,

subscapularis and infraspinatus contract and hold the head down in the glenoid. Rotation of the scapula is performed by courtesy of a muscular couple consisting of the upper fibres of trapezius, pulling upwards on the scapular spine, and serratus anterior pulling on the inferior angle.
[A:426; E:398; F:154]

237 The coracoclavicular ligament connects the clavicle to the coracoid process of the scapula. It consists of two parts—a flat quadrilateral trapezoid part and a thick triangular conoid part. It helps maintain the articulation of the weak acromioclavicular joint. Without its help, the clavicle dislocates superiorly and the scapula is displaced medially towards the midline.
[A:423; F:153]

238 The muscles associated with the intertubercular (bicipital) groove are the long head of biceps, latissimus dorsi, teres major and pectoralis major. As its name suggests, the groove is occupied by the tendon of the long head of biceps. On the lateral lip of the groove the pectoralis major is inserted. Medially the latissimus dorsi is inserted into the floor of the groove and teres major into the medial lip. There is a mnemonic for this which reinforces the above information: 'Lady Dee (latissimus dorsi) lies in bed between the two majors' (pectoralis major and teres major).
[A:325; H:96]

239 When considering the factors contributing to the stability of any joint it is as well to run through a 'check list' of structures which may be important. These are, first, bony articulations, second, ligaments (intrinsic or capsular and extrinsic or extracapsular) and, third, muscles. Applying this to the shoulder, it will be obvious that, unlike the hip, the ball-and-socket arrangement of the shoulder is very unstable, even allowing for the deepening effect of the glenoid socket by the cartilaginous labrum glenoidale. The capsule of the shoulder is lax, so the intrinsic (glenohumeral) ligaments must also be lax and therefore ineffective in preventing dislocation. The extrinsic coracoacromial ligament, however, forms an arch

above the joint, which prevents upward dislocation. The major factor in maintaining stability of the shoulder is the tonus of the muscles which act across it. These are the rotator cuff muscles (infraspinatus, supraspinatus, subscapularis and teres minor) which attach the humeral head to the scapula, and the long head of biceps which acts as a strong strap-like support over the head of the humerus. It should be said that these muscular supports are deficient inferiorly and it is in this direction that the humeral head usually dislocates. The shoulder joint pays for the large range of movement available to it by being rather unstable.
[A:424; F:155]

240   The rotator cuff muscles are the supraspinatus, infraspinatus, teres minor and subscapularis. They attach the scapula to the head of the humerus. Supraspinatus runs from the supraspinous fossa on the posterior aspect of the scapula to the upper facet of the greater tuberosity of the humerus. Infraspinatus arises from the infraspinous fossa and inserts onto the middle facet on the greater tuberosity. Supraspinatus and infraspinatus are supplied by the suprascapular nerve. Teres minor arises from the upper part of the lateral border of the scapula and inserts onto the lower facet. It is supplied by the axillary nerve. Subscapularis arises from the subscapular fossa on the anterior of the scapula. Whereas the other muscles run above or anterior to the shoulder and have a crowded insertion on the greater tuberosity, subscapularis runs posterior to the joint and is the only muscle to insert onto the lesser tuberosity. It is supplied by the subscapular nerves. The rotator cuff muscles are the major factor in determining the stability of the shoulder joint, and run anteriorly, superiorly and posteriorly to it. They are deficient inferiorly, which is the usual direction for shoulder dislocations to occur.
[A:425; C:202; E:396]

B   Applied answers

241   The effects of a partial or complete tear in the supraspinatus tendon is pain and spasm in the

middle range of abduction—60–120°. This is called the 'painful arc syndrome'. In a complete tear the patient cannot abduct the arm without shrugging the shoulder. Deltoid alone will not fully abduct the arm.
[F:158; H:114]

242 If the surgical neck is damaged or the shoulder dislocated, then the axillary nerve is endangered as it winds posteriorly from the brachial plexus to the deep side of the deltoid muscle. A damaged axillary nerve may result in a wasting of deltoid with a square-shaped shoulder as well as a small sensory loss on the upper lateral part of the arm.
[G:639; H:114]

243 The anatomical neck is the old epiphyseal plate and surrounds the smooth articular cartilage of the head of the humerus. The surgical neck, however, is some 2–3 cm below the head and greater tubercle and is the site of fracture during injury. It is the most superior part of the shaft.
[H:95]

244 A fall on an outstretched arm often causes this injury, which is one of the commonest sites of fracture in the body. The lateral fragment is depressed due to gravity and the weight of the limb but it is drawn medially and anteriorly by teres major, latissimus dorsi and, especially, pectoralis major. The eversion of the medial fragment is due to sternomastoid.
[D:182]

245 An axial x-ray in abduction is especially useful to demonstrate a dislocated shoulder.
[I:74; J:46]

C Information answers

246 This question is a little mean, as every student knows the axiom that 'veins are variable'. Nevertheless, in practice, the veins of the upper limb are used to take blood, to set up infusions and to pass long cannulae to the central veins and heart. The deep fascia separates the veins into a superficial network superficial to it and a deep network deep to it. The superficial veins

start in the dorsal plexus on the back of the hand. Two relatively constant veins ascend the arm from this point—the cephalic vein laterally and the basilic vein medially. The cephalic vein crosses the anatomical snuffbox, runs laterally up the forearm and arm, and then ascends in the furrow between the deltoid and pectoralis major muscles (deltopectoral groove). It pierces the clavipectoral fascia to drain into the axillary vein. The basilic vein runs up the medial side of the forearm. Halfway up the arm it pierces the deep fascia. At the lower border of teres major it becomes the axillary vein. There is usually a communication between the cephalic and basilic veins in the cubital fossa—the median cubital vein. The deep veins of the upper limb accompany the arteries in pairs as the venae comitantes. They drain to the venae comitantes of the brachial artery and from there to the axillary vein.
[A:699; G:64; J:204]

247   The median nerve is formed by two roots: a lateral root from the lateral cord of the brachial plexus and a medial root from the medial cord. Initially the nerve lies lateral to the brachial artery. However, halfway down the arm it crosses anterior to the artery to lie medial to it. In this position they descend together into the cubital fossa where they run deep to the bicipital aponeurosis (grâce à Dieu) fascia. The median nerve leaves the cubital fossa by passing between the two heads of pronator teres. The brachial artery divides near the apex of the cubital fossa into the radial and ulnar arteries. The ulnar artery passes deep to pronator teres to leave the cubital fossa; the radial artery leaves it by passing below brachioradialis.
[A:649, 1042; G:653; H:125]

248   Three nerves are related directly to the humerus at some point, and may be damaged by fractures at these points. The axillary nerve runs round the posterior part of the surgical neck of the humerus. Here it may be damaged by fractures or shoulder dislocations. The radial nerve runs round the spiral groove of the humeral shaft. The ulnar nerve runs posterior to the line of the elbow joint in a groove behind the medial humeral epicondyle.
[A:329; D:183]

249 The cephalic vein runs up the lateral aspect of the arm to enter the depression between the pectoralis major and deltoid muscles (deltopectoral groove). Here it pierces the clavipectoral fascia to enter the axillary vein.
[A:699; J:204]

250 When the elbow is fully extended and the hand supinated, the long axis of the ulna is not in a direct line with the long axis of the humerus but makes an angle with it. The forearm is angled laterally on the upper arm at an angle of about 160°—termed the carrying angle. It is caused by the fact that the medial lip of the trochlea extends further inferiorly than the lateral lip. The carrying angle is particularly marked in women.
[A:430]

251 The elbow can be divided into three subjoints, although they all share the same synovial cavity. First is the humeroulnar joint. This is the articulation between the trochlea of the humerus and the upper end of the ulna. It is here that flexion and extension occur. Second is the humeroradial joint. This is between the round capitulum of the humerus and the disc-shaped head of the radius. Third is the superior radioulnar joint. This is the articulation between the head of the radius and the radial notch on the ulna plus the annular ligament which runs round the radial head. The superior radioulnar joint and humeroradial joint allow the head of the radius to swivel against the capitulum. When transferred down the forearm this is converted into pronation and supination.
[A:429; G:659; H:122]

252 Pronation and supination occur about an axis which is a line drawn from the centre of the radial head to the base of the styloid process of the ulna. Pronation is brought about by pronator teres, running from the common flexor origin and ulna to a tubercle halfway down the radius, by pronator quadratus, joining the ulna and radius in the distal quarter, and by flexor carpi radialis. Supination occurs chiefly by courtesy of biceps which inserts on the posterior aspect of the radial tuberosity, thereby 'unwinding' the radius as it contracts, and to a

lesser extent by supinator running from the ulna and humerus posterior to the interosseous membrane and wrapping itself round the proximal part of the radius. They are aided by the two dorsal thumb muscles arising from the ulna, viz. extensor pollicis longus and abductor pollicis longus.
[A:434; E:451; F:166]

253 The ulnar nerve can normally be palpated as it passes in its groove behind the medial epicondyle. The superficial radial nerve can be palpated as it crosses the tendon of extensor pollicis longus on the dorsum of the wrist.
[A:1043, 1045; G:646, 686]

254 The cubital fossa is the area anterior to the elbow joint. It is triangular in shape with its base proximally and its apex directed distally. Its base is an imaginary line drawn between the two humeral epicondyles. Its lateral margin is formed by the brachioradialis muscle and the medial margin by pronator teres. They cross at the apex. The floor is composed of brachialis with a portion of supinator laterally. The roof is skin, superficial and deep fascia, the latter being reinforced medially by the bicipital aponeurosis. The fossa contains, from lateral to medial, the radial nerve, the biceps tendon, the brachial artery bifurcating into its two terminal branches, and the median nerve.
[A:650; G:655; H:125]

255 The anterior interosseous nerve is derived from the median nerve just proximal to pronator teres. It descends on the anterior aspect of the interosseous membrane with the anterior interosseous artery, between flexor pollicis longus laterally and flexor digitorum profundus medially. It ends on the carpus. It supplies the flexor pollicis longus, flexor digitorum profundus and pronator quadratus. It sends articular branches to the wrist, inferior radioulnar and carpal joints.

The posterior interosseous nerve arises from the radial nerve as it crosses the lateral humeral epicondyle. It runs through supinator, curving round the neck of the radius as it does so. It passes between the superficial and deep extensor muscles of the forearm, and at the lower

border of extensor pollicis brevis comes to lie on the posterior aspect of the interosseous membrane. It ends on the carpus. It supplies the extensor muscles of the forearm, wrist and carpal joints.
[A:1041, 1045; G:669; H:128]

256 The radial nerve is a branch of the posterior cord of the brachial plexus. It enters the posterior compartment of the arm with the profunda brachii artery between the long and medial heads of triceps, below teres major. It then enters the spiral groove between the lateral and medial heads of triceps. Here it is in direct continuity with the humerus and may be damaged by pressure or a fracture. In the groove it passes from the medial to the lateral side of the arm and eventually pierces the lateral intermuscular septum to enter the anterior compartment. It descends between brachialis medially and brachioradialis laterally to reach the cubital fossa.
[A:1044; G:640; H:118]

C Applied answers

257 The brachial artery is the direct continuation of the axillary artery distal to teres major muscle and lies medial to the upper humerus but winds anteriorly in front of brachialis to cross the elbow joint anteriorly between the humeral condyles. Its pulsations are palpable throughout its length as it descends the arm because it is only covered by skin and fascia. In the cubital fossa it is covered and protected by the bicipital aponeurosis which separates it from the numerous superficial veins of this region. Normally, it divides at the level of the elbow joint. However, it is the commonest large artery which is subject to anomalies such as high bifurcation, collateral vessels or a double artery which may envelop the median nerve.
[E:406; G:6119]

258 'Crutch palsy' is due to pressure on the radial nerve as it leaves the axilla. This results in an inability to form as tight a grip, as for this action both extensors (radial nerve) and flexors are required to form a tight power grip. This is an

example of synergism and can easily be demonstrated by trying to grip something very tightly with your wrist in full flexion. The wrist weakness will be due to loss of power in the finger and wrist extensors.
[C:255; D:211]

259 He has torn his biceps tendon, thus causing a large bulge of ruptured muscle fibres on his anterior arm. The pain is most likely referred to the shoulder joint and his difficulty in opening a door is due to the loss of biceps' two functions—elbow flexion and, in this case, more specifically supination.
[E:403]

260 This fracture results from a fall on the outstretched arm, and the seriousness of the injury depends on the degree of displacement anteriorly of the proximal humeral fragment. When the proximal fragment displaces, it may cause irritation or laceration of the brachial artery and median nerve. The loss of median nerve function may result in severely impaired pronation, reduced wrist flexion with ulnar deviation and, most drastically, the loss of thumb opposition as well as accompanying sensory deficits. In the long term, ischaemia due to interruption of the brachial artery may result in a Volkmann's contracture of the hand due to fibrosis of the long flexor and extensor muscles of the forearm. In this condition, the wrist is flexed and the metacarpophalangeal joints are extended whilst the interphalangeal joints flexed.
[G:653]

261 Division of the ulnar nerve at the elbow will cause only minimal sensory and vasomotor loss on the medial side of the hand and fingers. The resultant 'claw-hand' is due to paralysis of flexor digitorum profundus of the fourth and fifth fingers and all the intrinsic hand muscles. As these muscles atrophy, a 'guttered' look often appears between the metacarpals. Although there is a slight flexion deformity of the fourth and fifth fingers and the patient cannot abduct or adduct his fingers with his palm flat on the table, it is amazing how this injury may leave a reasonable functioning hand.
[D:212; E:421]

262 The child has a dislocated head of radius. This injury is seen most commonly in young children whose annular ligament of the radial head has not yet reached its normal configuration. In the adult it is cone-shaped, encircling the bulbous radial head, whereas in children it is a simple signet ring shape and the radial head is not developed, making it easy for a sudden pull to sublux the head out of the annular ligament. It is reduced by firm supination, screwing the radial head back into its anatomical position.
[G:659; H:122]

263 For a mainly right-handed population a right-handed thread means that supination is the action used to fix a screw. This is a strong movement using mainly the biceps muscle whereas the pronator teres and pronator quadratus, which are used in unscrewing, are not so powerful. A left-handed thread would reverse this situation.
[G:669]

264 'Miner's elbow' is in fact an olecranon bursitis due to the rubbing of the subcutaneous tissue overlying the olecranon whilst crawling down the pits or writing great volumes of work. It is a disease of enthusiastic authors!
[G:663]

265 There is normally a simple relationship between the epicondyles and the olecranon; in the extended elbow they lie on a straight line, whilst in the flexed elbow they form an equilateral triangle. If the elbow is dislocated these relationships will alter, whereas in a supracondylar fracture they remain constant.
[D:174; E:362]

266 The surgeon performs a transposition of the ulnar nerve, taking it from just posterior to the medial epicondyle and replacing it on the anterior aspect of the forearm. Thus usually solves the tingling problem but leaves the nerve relatively exposed to forearm injuries.
[G:664]

267 The bicipital aponeurosis or 'grâce à Dieu' fascia protects the median nerve and brachial artery from such incidents. The expanding mass is

therefore likely to be a haematoma or traumatic aneurysm of the brachial artery due to the student's not realising he had probed too deep.
[D:177; G:653; H:124]

268 Both palmaris longus and peroneus tertius are atavistic muscles not found in all of the population. Palmaris longus is missing in about 5–10 per cent of the population and in these people it is often easy to palpate the median nerve prior to its passing through the carpal tunnel.
[B:131; G:6124]

D Information answers

269 The common extensor origin gives rise to the five superficial extensor muscles of the forearm: extensor digiti minimi, extensor carpi ulnaris, extensor carpi radialis brevis and longus, extensor digitorum and anconeus. It is situated on the lateral epicondyle of the humerus.
[A:325; G:666; H:124]

270 The wrist joint is a synovial joint of the condyloid variety. The articular surfaces are formed by the scaphoid, lunate and triquetral bones distally. These form a convex ellipsoid mass which fits into a corresponding convex cavity proximally, formed by the lower end of the radius laterally and the articular disc medially. The ulna gives no contribution to the articular surface. The capsule is attached to the bones mentioned above and is reinforced laterally and medially to form the respective collateral ligaments. The movements permitted are flexion, extension, abduction and adduction (in combination, circumduction). Rotation cannot occur because the ellipsoid nature of the opposing surfaces prevents it. The function of rotation is taken over by pronation and supination.
[A:434; F:166]

271 Flexor carpi ulnaris (FCU) and flexor carpi radialis (FCR) pass anterior to the wrist joint on the ulnar and the radial aspect, respectively. Similarly, extensor carpi ulnaris (ECU) and extensor carpi radialis longus (ECRL) and brevis (ECRB) pass posterior to the wrist on their respective aspects of the joint. When the two flexors

contract together, flexion of the wrist results, and when the extensors contract, extension. If the ulnar flexor and ulnar extensor now contract, adduction of the wrist results. If the radial flexor and extensor are employed, abduction occurs. Therefore, the abductors of the wrist are FCR, ECRL and ECRB, and the adductors are FCU and ECU.
[A:438; D:196; F:170]

272 Muscles can only contract a certain proportion of their length. It follows that, if their origin and insertion are approximated by this amount, no further contraction can occur and their action will necessarily be weak. If the wrist is flexed, the long flexors of the finger work under this disadvantage and the resulting grip is weak. If, however, the wrist is extended prior to gripping, the origin and insertion the flexors are moved apart, the flexor muscles are stretched and the resulting grip will be powerful.
[A:438; E:457]

273 The anatomical snuffbox is situated on the lateral aspect of the wrist. It is bounded by the tendon of extensor pollicis longus posteriorly and the tendons of abductor pollicis longus and extensor pollicis brevis anteriorly. Its floor consists of the styloid process of the radius, the scaphoid bone, the trapezium and the base of the first metacarpal from proximal to distal. It contains the radial artery as it runs from the ventral to dorsal aspect of the wrist. The snuffbox is crossed by the cephalic vein and the cutaneous branches of the radial nerve.
[A:550; F:140; G:688; H:140]

D Applied answers

274 Because herpes zoster virus infection travels along a single nerve, it often demarcates the dermatomes. The C6 dermatome usually involves the lateral side of the forearm below the elbow and includes the thumb, thenar eminence and index finger. It does not cross the axial line and is always along the preaxial border of the arm, though, as with all dermatomes,

it is best defined by a smudge and not a definite clear line.
[E:470; G:541]

275 There is little difference in function between the ulnar nerve wrist and elbow injuries, but the wrist injury leaves the patient with a more pronounced claw on the medial fingers. This is due to the fact that the flexor digitorum profundus is not affected and thus causes a more pronounced claw. In an elbow injury to the ulnar nerve, this muscle is paralysed and the claw-hand is therefore less obvious. The sensory loss in both instances may be quite minimal and, surprisingly, it may be difficult to be sure that the nerve is damaged at all.
[D:212]

276 Other than the obvious cut muscle tendons, the two major nerves of the hand are both vulnerable. The median nerve lies just deep to palmaris longus and the ulnar nerve lies between the ulnar artery and pisiform bone. To test the ulnar nerve, the hand is placed palm downwards and the fingers abducted and adducted against resistance. To test the median nerve, the patient is asked to oppose the pulp of the thumb to the pulp of the little finger. Thumb opposition is impossible in median nerve lesions, as the thumb is laterally rotated and adducted and consequently looks like a monkey's or ape's hand.
[D:212; E:364]

277 Post-traumatic pain deep in the anatomical snuffbox is usually due to a fractured scaphoid bone. This often does not show up immediately, but after two weeks healing will be seen on an x-ray. Due to the blood supply arrangement this bone is a classic site of avascular necrosis.
[I:108; J:52]

278 Try this yourself and you will find that the power grip is very weak in acute wrist flexion. Normally, the wrist extensors work synergistically with the flexors of the fingers. Flexion of the wrist deprives the long flexor tendons of the ability to contract further and make a strong grip. Flexing the wrist will therefore make

someone relax his grip and drop whatever is in his hand.
[E:457]

E Information answers

279 The bones of the middle finger to be discussed will be the three phalanges (distal, middle and proximal) and the metacarpal. The muscles concerned are the long flexors, the extensor, the second lumbrical, the interossei and the adductor pollicis. The flexor digitorum profundus is inserted into the base of the distal phalanx. The flexor digitorum superficialis splits into two to allow the profundus to pass through it and is inserted into the base of the middle phalanx. The single extensor tendon is enlarged posterior to the metacarpophalangeal joint to form the extensor hood, which sends slips into the bases of all three phalanges. The lumbrical arises from the profundus tendon in front of the metacarpal and, passing lateral to the digit, is inserted into the extensor expansion. The middle finger's metacarpal has no palmar interosseous muscle attached to its anterior border but, instead, receives the transverse head of the adductor pollicis. Two dorsal interossei, however, insert onto the extensor expansion and base of the proximal phalanx of this digit, one on each side. They are bipennate muscles and arise from the adjacent borders of the second and third and third and fourth metacarpals. They move the middle finger either way in the coronal plane.
[A:546, 557; G:6106; H:145]

280 Where tendons run over bones they require lubrication by synovial sheaths. In the case of the long digital flexors of the hand, these conditions are met in the carpal tunnel and in the digits themselves. In the palm, the eight tendons of the flexor digitorum profundus and superficialis share a single sheath. The tendon of flexor pollicis longus has one of its own. Each digit of the hand possesses a digital synovial sheath for the profundus and superficialis tendons to that finger, the one to the little finger communicating with the palmar sheath. The flexor pollicis longus of the thumb has one of its

own which connects with the palmar sheath of that tendon.
[A:552; E:434]

281 The intrinsic muscles of the hand have their fleshy bellies actually in the hand, i.e. distal to the wrist joint. They are the palmaris brevis, the thenar and hypothenar muscles, adductor pollicis, the lumbricals and the palmar and dorsal interossei. They are supplied by the T1 root via the ulnar and median nerves.
[A:554; H:136]

282 The myotome of T1 is distributed to the small muscles of the hand. The T1 dermatome is along the medial side of the elbow and arm.
[A:1063, 1065; D:275; G:541]

283 The thenar muscles (flexor pollicis brevis, abductor pollicis brevis and opponens pollicis, but not adductor pollicis) are supplied by a branch of the median nerve which takes a recurrent and superficial course from the distal aspect of the flexor retinaculum to supply them. The hypothenar muscles are supplied by the deep branch of the ulnar nerve as it passes between the pisiform and the hook of the hamate. This nerve also usually innervates the adductor pollicis muscle.
[A:1043; E:437]

284 The interossei are of two sorts—palmar and dorsal. The palmar interossei arise from the metacarpal and are inserted into the dorsal expansion of the same digit. Those from the little and ring fingers arise from the radial aspect, that from the index finger from the ulnar aspect. The middle finger is deficient. The dorsal interossei are bipennate, arising from adjacent metacarpals to be inserted onto the extensor hood and the base of the proximal phalanges—the first two on the radial aspect of the index and middle fingers, the last two on the ulnar aspect of the middle and little fingers. The palmar interossei adduct the digits towards an imaginary axis along the middle finger; the dorsal interossei abduct them. The dorsal interossei to the middle finger (axis) can move it either way. Together, they flex the metacarpophalangeal joints and extend the interphalan-

geal joints by virtue of their insertion into the extensor hood.

The lumbricals arise from the flexor digitorum profundus tendons, adjacent to the bases of the metacarpals, and, passing laterally along their respective digits, are inserted into the extensor hood. They flex the metacarpophalangeal joints but, by pulling on the extensor hood, extend the interphalangeal joints.

Failure of these muscles results in inability to extend the interphalangeal joints while keeping the metacarpophalangeal joints flexed, a movement essential in writing.
[A:554; E:440]

285 The ulnar and radial arteries anastomose in the palm to form a superficial and a deep palmar arch.

The superficial arch is formed mainly by the ulnar artery. It curves across the palm deep to the palmar aponeurosis, level with the distal border end of the fully extended thumb. It sends digital branches (two to each digit, one on each side) to the medial three and one-half digits (little, ring, middle and half the index fingers). The radial artery passes across the snuffbox to the dorsum of the hand, and re-enters the palm by diving through the first interosseous space, to give the main input to the deep palmar arch. It runs across the palm anterior to the metacarpals and interossei at a more proximal level than the superficial arch, being level with the proximal border of the extended thumb. The deep branch of the ulnar nerve lies within its curve. It supplies the lateral one and a half digits (thumb and half of the index finger) by digital branches. These branches are named the arteria radialis indicis and the arteria princeps pollicis.
[A:653, 655; J:178]

286 The superficial lymph vessels of the upper limb follow the cephalic vein laterally and basilic vein medially. The former end in the infraclavicular nodes of the deltopectoral groove. The latter pass through the epitrochlear node as the basilic vein pierces the deep fascia half-way up the arm, and end in the lateral axillary nodes around the axillary vein. The deep lymph of the arm also passes to these nodes. The lateral

nodes in turn drain to the apical axillary lymph nodes.
[A:732; I:121]

287 The thumb is set at right angles to the other digits. Its movements are therefore expressed differently from those of the other digits and this leads to confusion. When discussing the movements of the digits, a line should be drawn in the plane of the nail of the digit concerned. Movement towards the pulp of the digit is flexion, and towards the nail is extension. Movements in the plane of the nail are abduction and adduction. In the case of the thumb, abduction brings the whole digit anteriorly in the anatomical position; movement posteriorly is adduction. Flexion of the thumb at the carpometacarpal joint is associated with medial rotation. In this way the pulp of the thumb is brought into apposition with the pulp of another digit. This is termed opposition. Extension is similarly associated with lateral rotation.
[A:439; E:455; F:133]

E Applied answers

288 Wrist drop is the most noticeable injury, due to loss of all finger and wrist extensors. This also considerably weakens the power grip. The sensory loss, however, is often only very limited due to overlap of the nerves' sensory distribution but may include a strip down the posterior aspect of arm and forearm as well as a small area of anaesthesia over the first dorsal interosseus muscle.
[C:255; D:212]

289 The median nerve lesion is the most disabling because thumb opposition is lost, as well as the sensation over the thumb, index and middle fingers. Consequently, all fine pincer movements such as writing are almost impossible.
[D:212; E:454]

290 Dupuytren's contracture is due to fibrosis within the palmar aponeurosis causing flexion of the metacarpophalangeal and proximal interphalangeal joints, especially in the ring and

little fingers. The distal interphalangeal joint is not affected, as the palmar aponeurosis inserts only into the middle and proximal phalanges.
[D:214; G:666; H:131]

291 The small muscles of the thumb are all innervated by the median nerve, which has to pass through the carpal tunnel below the flexor retinaculum. The skin above the muscles, however, is supplied by the superficial palmar branch of the median nerve, and this branches off just proximal to the retinaculum and thus escapes compression.
[G:674; H:131]

292 The long flexor tendons of the thumb are surrounded by synovial sheaths. An infection in the pulp might readily spread proximally where, in some people, it joins the ulnar bursa, both of them passing deep to the retinaculum and extending for 2–3 cm to the level of the wrist.
[D:215; E:434]

293 Guttering of the dorsum of the hand is seen in atrophy of the interossei. Froment's sign is seen when a patient is asked to grip a piece of paper between thumb and index finger, and, due to adductor pollicis paralysis, the patient compensates by visibly contracting flexor pollicis longus instead of adducting the thumb. Clawed ring and little fingers, as with the other signs, would suggest an ulnar nerve lesion.
[C:294; D:212; E:476]

294 This operation is referred to as a cervical sympathectomy, when in fact it is an upper thoracic sympathectomy performed through an incision in the neck. Cutting the sympathetic chain below the T3 ganglion, one tries not to touch T1 as this may result in a Horner's syndrome. The removal of T2–4 sympathetic segments removes control of sweating and vasoconstriction and, hopefully, results in a warmed dry hand, instead of the painfully cold sweating hand seen in Raynaud's disease.
[D:328; E:793]

THORAX

A Information answers

295 In the upper part of the thorax, during inspiration, the first rib remains relatively fixed. Owing to the anteroinferior slope of the ribs, contraction of the external intercostal muscles forces the sternum forwards and upwards like the handle of a pump, thus increasing the anteroposterior diameter of the thorax.

In the area of the lower ribs, contraction of the external intercostals raises the centre of the ribs as one would lift the handle of a bucket, thereby increasing the transverse thoracic diameter.
[A:514; B:276; E:77]

296 The following 'events' occur at the plane of T4:
   1 – Manubriosternal joint (angle of Louis)
   2 – Beginning and end of aortic arch
   3 – Bifurcation of trachea
   4 – Junction of superior and inferior mediastinum
   5 – Second costosternal joint
   6 – Confluence of vena azygos with superior vena cava
   7 – Thoracic duct runs from right to left
   8 – Ligamentum arteriosum lies on this plane
[A:1195; E:1; I:663]

297 The external intercostal muscles would be used during inspiration. Contraction of any intercostal muscle shortens the intercostal space. If this is associated with fixation of the first rib, elevation of all the other ribs will occur, with an increase in transverse and anteroposterior thoracic diameters. The anteroinferior direction of the external intercostal fibres aids this lifting action. Contraction of the intercostal muscles also prevents the intercostal spaces from being 'sucked in' as the negative intrathoracic pressure increases during inspiration.
[A:514; C:497; E:54; F:397]

298 The interspace is supplied with arterial blood from a single posterior intercostal artery (a branch of the descending thoracic aorta) and two anterior intercostal arteries (branches of the

144

internal thoracic artery). These all anastomose within the interspace. The veins run with the arteries to the internal thoracic and hemiazygos veins. The above vessels run in the plane between the internal and innermost intercostal muscles, incompletely guarded by the subcostal groove.
[A:657; B:268; E:55; F:398]

299   The intercostal nerves are the anterior primary rami of the first eleven thoracic spinal nerves. They run in their respective intercostal spaces between the internal and innermost intercostal muscles. Their branches are the collateral branch which runs at a lower level than the main nerve, a lateral cutaneous branch and an anterior cutaneous branch at its termination. The nerves are motor to the intercostal muscles and sensory to the ribs, joints, skin and pleura or peritoneum associated with their intercostal space.
[A:1048; B:270; E:55; F:398]

300   The lower five pairs of ribs are 'false ribs'; that is, they do not articulate directly with the sternum. The eleventh and twelfth ribs have no anterior articulation and are the 'floating ribs'. The eighth, ninth and tenth pairs are attached to each other via their costal cartilages, forming the costal margins.
[A:251; B:260; C:493; G:11]

301   There are two articulations with the vertebral column.
      In the costovertebral joint, the head of the rib articulates via synovial joints with the bodies of T6 and T5 and via a ligament with the intervening disc.
      In the costotransverse joint; the tubercle of the rib articulates with the right transverse process of T6 via a synovial joint; it is strengthened by associated ligaments which are the two from the transverse processes of T6 (costotransverse ligament and lateral costotransverse ligament) and one to the transverse process of T5 (superior costotransverse ligament).
[A:418; B:275; E:52; F:395; G:531]

A   Applied answers

302   These three points are all bony landmarks so they are relatively consistent at T2, T4/5 and T7

vertebral levels, respectively. The manubrio-sternal joint is also called the sternal angle (Louis). It is an important landmark for counting ribs, as the second costal cartilage articulates laterally at this joint. In most normal adults it is fairly easy to palpate and is thus commonly used by clinicians as a reference point.
[D:1; E:43; H:152]

303 Lymph from all of the skin and superficial fasciae of the back and abdomen above the level of the umbilicus and iliac crests drains to the axillary group of lymph nodes. Structures in the skin of the chest drain to the anterior axillary nodes, and a melanoma of the back would drain to the posterior axillary lymph nodes. These are found around the subscapular vessels lying on subscapularis muscle and are consequently often termed the subscapular group of axillary lymph nodes. Metastases might spread from this group to the central groups of nodes, in the axillary fat, and eventually to the apical nodes which lie on the axillary vein between pectoralis minor and the clavicle.
[E:62; F:87]

304 The level of the umbilicus is a watershed for lymphatic drainage of the skin of the anterior abdominal wall, so a truly paraumbilical tattoo will drain both above and below this watershed. In practice, this means that both right and left anterior axillary nodes as well as both groups of superficial inguinal nodes are likely to be affected.
[E:62; H:109, 207]

305 However effective a single spinal nerve block is, it is most unlikely to cause any sensory loss because the overlap between contiguous dermatomes is quite considerable. In fact, each segmental nerve overlaps its neighbour to such a degree that, unless at least two consecutive dorsal roots are anaesthetised, no sensory loss is apparent. The dermatomes for pain and temperature are very similar, but those of touch tend to be more extensive. It would be more appropriate if textbook diagrams did not show dermatomes between lines but between thick smudges!
[D:205; G:541]

306 Tuberculosis of a vertebral body may indeed be painful but one would at first expect that pathology of T9 vertebral body would give thoracic pain posteriorly. The patient's acute abdominal pain is explained by the fact that the pain is referred to the longest fibres of the spinal nerves involved. The T9 spinal nerve has its anterior cutaneous branches in the skin between the xiphoid process and the umbilicus. It is here that referred pain from the back may be felt.
[E:55; G:117; H:204]

307 Shingles is the term used to describe a herpes zoster infection. This tends to pick a single nerve, often a mixed spinal nerve or a branch of the trigeminal nerve in the face, and the classic sign of this disease is a vesicular rash along the distribution of that nerve. In this way it maps out the dermatomes. The skin around the umbilicus is suppled by T10 spinal nerve and, more specifically, by its anterior cutaneous branches.
[E:37; G:25; H:204]

308 This narrowing of the aorta usually occurs in the vicinity of the ductus arteriosus, which may be still patent. In adult coarctation the collateral circulation usually includes branches of the subclavian artery such as the internal thoracic, transverse cervical and transverse scapular as well as the intercostal arteries. Some vessels of the thoracic inlet such as the vertebral and anterior spinal arteries are also involved. After some time this collateral circulation, especially around the intercostal arteries, may be visible on a plain chest x-ray as notching of the inferior border of the ribs. This is usually seen in older children and adults and is due to the erosion of the ribs by tortuous dilated intercostal arteries.
[E:39, 64; H:195]

309 Interchondral joints in the lower thoracic region are prone to subluxation, especially following trauma. The eighth, ninth and tenth costal cartilages may be involved, and it is extremely easy to trap the intercostal nerve when the costal margin 'clicks' out of place. This may cause stimulation of the intercostal nerve and hence spontaneous contraction of its myotome. In the case of the ninth intercostal nerve this

will cause contraction of the three sheet-like abdominal muscles, viz. external and internal obliques and transversus abdominis. It will also cause a segment of the rectus abdominis to contract just superior to the umbilicus. This clinical problem of interchondral subluxation is often misdiagnosed as cardiac or upper abdominal pathology, when careful examination will reveal a 'clicking rib' or 'clicking costa'.
[G:117; H:155]

310 The first rib is the shortest, widest, strongest and flattest as well as having the most acute curve of all the ribs. Its costochondral articulation lies just below and lateral to the sternoclavicular joint and, radiologically, looks as if it is broken off at this point, especially if seen in a posteroanterior view of thorax. The costochondral joint of the first rib is also often visible on an oblique view of the sternum.
[H:151; I:714; J:68]

311 Cervical ribs occur in about 0.5 per cent of the population and are often bilateral. Though previously thought to be the cause of 'cervical rib syndrome' or 'scalenus anterior syndrome', it is now evident that the general term of 'thoracic outlet syndrome' is more appropriate—some of these people having no cervical ribs. The essential symptom of these syndromes is involvement of the lower trunk of the brachial plexus. In those without a rib, this may be caused by the neurovascular bundle being trapped between the first rib and clavicle or by a fibrous band from C7 to the first rib. The symptoms include tingling, numbness and even pain in the distribution of the T1 dermatome, which lies along the medial border of the forearm. Vascular changes and wasting of the intrinsic muscles of the hand may also accompany this neurological deficit.
[E:63; G:17]

312 The body of the sternum is formed from four sternebrae which ossify from either single or bilateral centres, usually during the last few months of intrauterine life. Fusion normally takes place from below upwards between the seventh and fifteenth years. So, if three separate sternebrae are visible, one would think of a

child of that age. By 25 years the body is unified, and in some 10 per cent of people the manubriosternal joint is fused after the age of 30.

[C:496; G:16; H:150; I:632]

B Information answers

313 The surface marking of the dome of the pleura is a curved line, convex upwards, drawn from the sternoclavicular joint to the junction of the medial and middle thirds of the clavicle. The highest point of the line is 2.5 cm above the clavicle.

[A:1192; B:706; D:2; F:402; G:124; H:152]

314 The parietal pleura is supplied by somatic nerves and is therefore sensitive to pain. The costal part is supplied by the relevant intercostal nerves. The diaphragmatic part is supplied by the phrenic nerve centrally and the lowest intercostal nerves peripherally. The mediastinal portion is also supplied by the phrenic nerve.

In contrast, the visceral pleura is supplied by autonomic fibres and is insensitive to pain.

[A:1194; B:284; E:70]

315 The pulmonary ligament is situated at the root of the lung where the visceral and parietal layers of pleura meet as a sleeve surrounding the structures passing to and from the lung. This sleeve hangs down inferiorly as the pulmonary ligament. It is supposed to expand to allow movements of the lung root and expansion of the pulmonary veins.

[A:1198; E:72; G:128]

316 The pleural cavity is the space between the parietal and visceral layers of pleura. It is normally collapsed and contains only a few millilitres of lubricant fluid but may become abnormally distended with air or fluid.

[A:1191; B:284; E:70; F:401]

317 The lymph vessels travel along the bronchi to the hila of the lungs, filtering en route through many lymph nodes within the lung substance. There are numerous lymph nodes at the lung root (tracheobronchial nodes). The lymph

drains superiorly from these nodes as the bronchomediastinal trunk, one on each side of the body, which ascend adjacent to the trachea and end in the thoracic duct on the left and in the right lymphatic duct on the right.
[A:744; B:329]

318 The lungs do not completely fill the pleural cavity but leave recesses where two layers of parietal pleura are in apposition. The costodiaphragmatic recess is found posteriorly and laterally where the pleura covering the diaphragm is in contact with that covering the ribs. The costomediastinal recess is situated between the mediastinal pleura and that covering the adjacent left border of the sternum and ribs. Its presence is due to a deficiency of the left lung in this area, termed the cardiac notch.
[A:1193; B:287; E:45]

319 Each main bronchus divides into lobar bronchi. These each divide again to form segmental bronchi. The part of each lobe supplied by one of these tertiary bronchi is a bronchopulmonary segment.
[A:1187; F:412; G:142; H:176]

320 The middle lobe of the right lung is situated in the anteroinferior part of the right thoracic space between the oblique and transverse fissures. The oblique fissure runs in an oblique line from the spine of T3 to the sixth costochondral junction. The transverse fissure runs from the right fourth costochondral junction to the oblique fissure which it meets in the mid-axillary line.

The right middle lobe corresponds to the lingula of the upper lobe on the left.
[A:1197; B:292; E:74; H:154]

321 The bronchial arteries are usually branches of the descending thoracic aorta. They vary in number—normally there is one on the right and two on the left. They anastomose to some extent with the pulmonary arteries.

Some of the bronchial venous blood passes to the pulmonary veins and thence to the left atrium. The remainder forms bronchial veins which drain, on the right, into the azygos vein

and, on the left, to the superior intercostal or
hemiazygos vein.
[A:1204; H:185]

B Applied answers

322 Pleurisy is inflammation of the pleurae but
causes little discomfort if only the visceral
pleura is involved because this is insensitive to
pain and touch due to its autonomic innervation. However, the parietal pleura is supplied
by the intercostal nerves (costal pleura), phrenic
nerves (mediastinal and central diaphragmatic
pleura) and the lower five or six intercostal
nerves (peripheral diaphragmatic pleura). The
regions supplied by the lower intercostal nerves
may present as referred pain to the dermatomes
of the upper abdomen and may therefore be
indistinguishable from the pain of gastrointestinal origin.
[B:284; F:417]

323 The consequences obvious to the patient are
often severe sharp pain, but in anatomical
terms the important fact is that the pleural
cavity is now opened and air can rush in,
causing a pneumothorax with collapse of the
lung involved.
[B:286]

324 A pleural effusion is a collection of excess fluid
within the pleural cavity. Normally this contains only a thin film of pleural fluid, which is
just enough to act as a lubricant for the opposing visceral and parietal layers. The exact position of this fluid will depend on gravity and the
posture of the patient. In bed-ridden patients it
tends to collect at the base of the lungs, especially posteriorly where it is easily detected by
percussion.
[E:54]

325 A pneumothorax may be drained with the aid
of a catheter and an underwater seal apparatus
at one of two commonly chosen sites. These are
the second intercostal space in the mid-
clavicular line and the fifth or sixth intercostal
space in the mid-axillary line. In the anterior
approach the trocar and cannula pass through

the anaesthetised skin, superficial fascia, pectoralis major and minor before penetrating the intercostal muscle fibres. Immediately deep to the thin membrane of the innermost intercostal muscle is the parietal pleura, which acts as the external limit of a pneumothorax. The more lateral approach is preferred by patients because the pectoral muscles are not involved, thus giving pain-free movement of the arm.
[B:286; E:54]

326 The cervical pleura resembles a dome extending from the junction of the medial and middle thirds of the clavicle to the sternoclavicular joint. The highest point of the dome lies some 2.5 cm above the clavicle and the apex projects into the base of the neck. In this region, the pleural fascia is thickened to support the pleura and is known as the suprapleural membrane (Sibson's fascia). The veins used for catheterisation in the neck include the internal jugular, subclavian and brachiocephalic veins. The internal jugular vein drains blood from the brain and superficial parts of the face, and its surface marking is a band from the earlobe to the medial end of the clavicle. The subclavian vein is a continuation of the axillary and begins at the outer border of the first rib. It unites with the internal jugular vein just behind the sternoclavicular joint, thus forming the brachiocephalic vein. All the above veins are immediate anterior relations of the cervical pleural domes, as many an inexperienced physician has found on performing a central venous catheterisation! Pneumothorax, haemothorax and even chylothorax are complications of this procedure, particularly after using the subclavian route.
[G:941; H:109, 191]

327 It is prudent to avoid performing a left subclavian or brachiocephalic puncture due to the presence of the thoracic duct terminating in the angle between the internal jugular and subclavian veins. If at the same time as damaging the thoracic duct near its termination one lacerates the cervical pleura, a chylothorax can result.
[G:941; H:191]

328 The apicoposterior bronchus is found in the left upper lobe and is seen especially well on a left

lateral or right anterior oblique bronchogram. There is considerable variation in bronchopulmonary segmentation, therefore bronchography is a less reliable method of correct identification than anatomical sectioning. However, the apicoposterior segmental bronchus quickly further divides into the separate apical and posterior segments.
[H:181; I:605; J:160]

329 The surface markings of the apical basal segment are fairly similar in both lungs, the superior limit of this bronchopulmonary segment being the oblique fissure posteriorly. The apex and upper border of this segment therefore lie along a line joining the spine of T3 and descending obliquely to follow the line of the sixth rib to the sixth costochondral junction. With the arm raised above the head, this lies along the medial border of the rotated scapula. The segment of lung tissue is a pyramid whose apex is along this line and whose base is about the area of the palm placed on the back just lateral to erector spinae. The apical basal segment is also called the superior basal or lower lobe segment.
[H:153, 181]

330 The basic principle of effective postural drainage is positioning the patient so that secretions will drain from the diseased segment with the aid of gravity. The addition of a physiotherapist's skills has been likened to the attempts to extract the last drop of ketchup from a tomato sauce bottle by hitting the base whilst pointing the neck of the bottle downwards. Basal segments, therefore, may require the patient to be tipped head downwards and, in the specific case of a posterior basal segment, in a prone position.
[A:1189; H:183]

331 An apical carcinoma often affects structures which lie in direct contact with the suprapleural membrane (Sibson's fascia). These include the sympathetic trunk, the cervicothoracic or stellate ganglion, and the roots of T1. Invasion of the sympathetic pathways at this level may cause a Horner's syndrome due to the interruption of the sympathetic supply to the head and neck. This syndrome consists of a constricted

153

pupil, flushed and dry skin of the face, drooping of the upper eyelid (ptosis) and retraction of the eyeball (enophthalmos). The drooped upper lid is due to partial paralysis of levator palpebrae superioris, whose superior tarsal portion of smooth muscle (Müller) is innervated by sympathetic fibres from the cervical chain. The pain in the little finger may be caused by direct involvement of the T1 nerve, whose dermatome lies along the medial border of the forearm and hand.

[C:501; E:57; G:148; H:190]

C Information answers

332 The conducting tissue of the heart consists of specialised cardiac muscle. The sinuatrial (SA) node is the pacemaker. It is situated in the upper part of the sulcus terminalis superior to the opening of the superior vena cava into the right atrium. From here the impulse spreads over the atria to reach the atrioventricular (AV) node. This structure is found in the lower part of the interatrial septum, next to the septal cusp of the tricuspid valve. From here the impulse spreads down the atrioventricular bundle, which forms the only electrical and muscular continuity between the atria and ventricles. Where the interventricular septum becomes muscular the bundle divides into two—right and left. The right bundle runs down the right-hand side of the septum and crosses the right ventricle as the moderator band. The left bundle divides again and the two terminal branches run down the left side of the septum. All the bundles terminate in the ventricles as a subendocardial plexus of conducting tissue.

[A:611; B:315; E:85; F:435; G:166]

333 Most of the venous blood of the heart drains into the coronary sinus. This structure runs in the coronary sulcus on the posterior aspect of the heart and drains into the right atrium. It receives, first, the great cardiac vein which ascends in the anterior interventricular groove to reach the coronary sulcus, second, the middle cardiac vein which ascends in the posterior interventricular groove and, third, the small cardiac vein which accompanies the marginal

branch of the right coronary artery along the inferior border of the heart. It also receives the oblique vein which lies behind the left atrium and the posterior ventricular veins which drain the diaphragmatic surface.

The rest of the venous blood either drains directly into the heart chambers via the venae cordis minimae (Thebesian veins) or reaches the right atrium directly via anterior cardiac veins which run across the front of the right ventricle.
[A:685; B:316; E:89; G:159; H:171]

334 The coronary arteries are thus named because they run in the coronary sulcus. This was originally in the coronal plane but has rotated during development to lie more in the sagittal plane.
[A:618; B:316; E:89; G:159; H:166]

335 The left coronary artery arises from the left posterior aortic sinus. It runs forwards for 1 cm between the pulmonary trunk and the left atrial appendage, where it divides into the anterior descending and circumflex branches. The former runs down the interventricular groove on the front of the heart. The latter continues in the coronary sulcus onto the posterior aspect of the heart, where it anastomoses with the right coronary artery.

There is much individual variation in the distribution of the coronary arteries. The left usually supplies the anterior part of the interventricular septum and adjacent portions of the right ventricle. It supplies the entire left ventricle except for a small strip on its diaphragmatic surface. It also supplies the posterior aspect of the left atrium.
[A:618; B:317; E:89; G:157; H:166]

336 The margins of the cusps of the atrioventricular valves are connected by tendinous cords (chordae tendineae) to muscular projections of the apical part of the ventricular wall (papillary muscles). During ventricular systole the papillary muscles contract and, by pulling on the chordae tendineae, draw the cusps together. This prevents the cusps being forced into the atria during systole, thereby maintaining the competence of the valve.
[A:604; B:310; E:86; G:167; H:163]

337 The right atrium receives the superior vena
cava, the inferior vena cava and the coronary
sinus, which drain the upper parts of the body,
the lower parts and the heart, respectively. It
also receives its share of minute heart veins
(venae cordis minimae) and one or two anterior
cardiac veins.
[A:601; B:310; E:83; F:430]

338 There are three layers in the pericardium: an
outer fibrous layer and two inner serous layers.
The outer serous layer is the parietal pericardium which is closely adherent to the fibrous
layer. The inner serous layer is the visceral
pericardium (epicardium) which closely invests
the heart. The pericardial cavity, containing a
few millilitres of lubricant fluid, is found between the two serous layers.
[A:597; B:303; F:420]

339 The phrenic nerves are embedded in the fibrous
pericardium. They innervate this structure with
sensory fibres. They also supply the parietal
serous pericardium in a similar fashion. The
outer layers of the pericardium are therefore
supplied by somatic nerves and are sensitive to
pain.
[A:598; G:146]

340 The transverse sinus of the pericardium is
found at the base of the pericardial cavity. It is a
passage which exists between the reflections of
pericardium around the arterial pole (aorta and
pulmonary trunk) and venous pole (pulmonary
veins and venae cavae). It is the remains of a
hole which appears in the dorsal mesocardium
during development.

The oblique sinus of the pericardium is found
posterior to the heart. It is a recess shaped like
three sides of a square, open inferiorly, and is
formed by the reflection of the pericardium
round the venous pole (pulmonary veins and
venae cavae). This part of the pericardial cavity
sits between the left atrium anteriorly and the
oesophagus posteriorly.
[A:598; B:304; E:83; G:161]

341 The right and left phrenic nerves are embedded
in the fibrous pericardium together with their
accompanying blood vessels (pericardiophrenic

artery and veins). The central tendon of the diaphragm and the fibrous pericardium are fused. The phrenic nerves supply both the pericardium and diaphragm.
[A:1195; G:146]

C Applied answers

342 The heart valves lie on an approximate diagonal line from the third left costosternal joint to the fifth or sixth right costosternal junction. Along this imaginary line across the body of the sternum they are arranged from superior to inferior in the following order—pulmonary, aortic, mitral and tricuspid. To hear the sounds of these valves closing during the cardiac cycle, one listens to where the sound is transmitted along the vessel through which the blood flows after passing through the valve; for example, the aortic sound is heard best in the right second intercostal space anterior to the ascending aorta. The mitral valve is usually heard best in the region of the apex beat.
[B:313; E:91; H:152]

343 The right heart shadow is formed from above downwards by the right brachiocephalic vein, superior vena cava, right atrium and inferior vena cava. The left heart border is formed from the aortic knuckle, pulmonary trunk, auricular appendage of the left atrium and left ventricle.
[D:53; I:714; J:58]

344 The heart is an internal organ and hence its sensory innervation is experienced as referred pain to its dermatomes. Because the heart is innervated bilaterally, and the sensory input from the heart is via the upper four or five thoracic dorsal roots, the pain of myocardial infarction is usually a crushing band-like vise in the T1–4 dermatomes and may also radiate along the medial side of the arm (normally left) and into the jaw and lower neck. Pain located in the region of the apex beat is normally of chest wall or supratentorial origin!
[A:1075; D:328; F:436]

345 The foramen ovale is the passage through which fetal blood passes from the right to the

left atrium. In about 75 per cent of adults it is completely obliterated, i.e. the septum primum and septum secundum are fused. In 25 per cent of individuals there is an overlap of the two septa, thus giving a physiologically normal person showing an apparently normal fossa ovalis; however, on detailed post-mortem examination there is no fusion and a probe or finger can pass through the still patent foramen ovale. Failure of any septal overlap will lead to a patent foramen ovale and an atrioseptal defect (ASD).
[A:153; F:431]

346 The right ventricle is the anterior chamber of the heart which would be lacerated in this case. Remember that the right inferior border on a chest x-ray is the right atrium and the left atrium is the posterior chamber of the heart. The apex beat is where the right ventricle anteriorly and left ventricle posteriorly are felt as one pulsation on the chest wall. Classically, it is in the left fifth intercostal space along the mid-clavicular line, or about 9 cm from the midline.
[D:30; G:153; H:160]

347 Examination of the coronary arteries is nowadays a routine procedure, and, using selective arteriograms, the right and left coronary arteries can be seen individually. A right selective coronary arteriogram would normally reveal branches to the sinuatrial node as well as the atrioventricular node.
[H:167; I:754; J:166]

348 A lateral view of the lower oesphagus during a barium swallow will normally reveal three indentations of its anterior border: superiorly lies the arch of the aorta, then the indentation due to the left main bronchus and inferiorly the indentation due to the left atrium. A patient with mitral valve disease may present with left atrial hypertrophy which can often be seen on the barium swallow.
[B:282; I:724; J:234]

349 The inner surfaces of both auricular appendages are rough and ridged by the musculi pectinati. The right atrium itself is divided by a ridge, the crista terminalis, anterior to which the atrial wall is rough and covered in musculi

pectinati whilst posteriorly the atrium is smooth. This is because the right atrium developed from the primitive sinus venosus (smooth) and primitive atrium (trabeculated musculi pectinati). Sometimes a faint groove can be seen on the exterior of the atrium, corresponding to the crista, and is termed the sulcus terminalis.
[F:430; G:163; H:162]

350 The left costoxiphoid approach to the pericardial cavity is often chosen, as this site tends to avoid the lungs and pleurae, due to the presence of the cardiac notch, and it is well away from the major coronary arteries. The needle is inclined superiorly and posteriorly at 45° to the patient's transverse plane and angled slightly medially to avoid the superior epigastric vessels running in the posterior rectus sheath. Having pierced the skin and superficial fascia, the needle passes through the anterior rectus sheath and left rectus abdominis muscle. The needle next encounters transversus abdominis, which forms the muscular posterior rectus sheath, and, after sliding over the superior surface of the diaphragm, passes through the fibrous and parietal serous pericardia. The tip of the needle will now lie between the parietal and visceral serous pericardium and hence in the cavity containing an effusion.
[E:115; G:151]

D Information answers

351 The mediastinum is arbitrarily divided into superior and inferior by a horizontal line through the sternal angle (T4). The inferior mediastinum is further subdivided into anterior, middle and posterior mediastina—the contents of the pericardium forming the middle mediastinum—the anterior mediastinum being anterior to the pericardium and the posterior mediastinum posterior. The anterior mediastinum therefore lies below T4 and between sternum and pericardium. The anterior mediastinum contains the inferior part of the thymus gland, fat, some lymph nodes and the sternopericardial ligaments.
[A:1195; B:278; D:29; E:68; F:400]

352   The thoracic duct commences in the abdomen at the superior end of the cisterna chyli. It enters the abdomen in company with the aorta on the right side of that vessel to lie on the right of the oesophagus. It ascends the posterior mediastinum, passing behind the oesophagus and reaching its left side at T4. It runs superiorly in this position into the neck. It passes laterally behind the carotid sheath and then arches forwards over the dome of the pleura to drain into the confluence of the left subclavian and left internal jugular veins.
[A:727; D:47; G:183]

353   The splanchnic nerves arise from the lower ganglia of the thoracic sympathetic trunk: the greater splanchnic nerve from ganglia 5–9, the lesser splanchnic nerve from ganglia 10 and 11 and the least splanchnic nerve from ganglion 12. These greater and lesser nerves pierce the crura of the diaphragm from medial to lateral, respectively. The greater and lesser nerves end in the coeliac ganglion on their respective sides. The least nerve runs behind the medial arcuate ligament and ends in the corresponding renal plexus.

    These nerves contain preganglionic sympathetic fibres.
[A:1074; B:335; F:480; G:147]

354   The transversely running structures in the mediastinum pass external to (i.e. behind) structures running vertically. Thus, for instance, the hemiazygos veins pass behind the descending aorta.
[A:1195; F:445]

355   For the purpose of description, the oesophagus is divided into upper, middle and lower thirds.

    The upper third is supplied by branches of the inferior thyroid arteries; the middle third by branches of the descending thoracic aorta; the lower third by branches of the left gastric artery.

    The veins from the upper third run to the inferior thyroid veins, from the middle third to the azygos system and from the lower third to the left gastric vein, which is a tributary of the portal vein. Thus the venous blood from the upper two-thirds runs to systemic veins, and from the lower third to portal veins. The lower

end of the oesophagus is therefore a site of portosystemic anastomosis.
[A:1254; E:100; G:184]

356 The white rami communicantes comprise the total afferent supply to the sympathetic chains. They are found only between T1 and L2, running from the mixed spinal nerve to the sympathetic chain. They contain preganglionic sympathetic fibres whose cell bodies are in the lateral horns of the spinal cord. They are white because they are myelinated.

The grey rami communicantes are found throughout the spinal cord and comprise only part of the efferents of the sympathetic chain. They contain postganglionic sympathetic fibres and run from the sympathetic chain to the spinal nerve. Being devoid of a myelin sheath, they are grey.
[A:1068; B:335; C:58; E:27; F:45]

357 The lowest cervical and the uppermost thoracic ganglion of the sympathetic chain are frequently fused to form the stellate ganglion. This is found anterior to the neck of the first rib and behind the origin of the vertebral artery.
[A:1073; B:785; G:946]

358 The superior mediastinum is bounded by the manubrium anteriorly, the bodies of the first four thoracic vertebrae posteriorly and the upper parts of the two lungs laterally. It consists of loose connective tissue in which various structures are embedded. From anterior to posterior, these are: thymus gland, the great veins and the superior vena cava of which they are tributaries, the aortic arch and its branches (the great arteries), the trachea, the oesophagus and thoracic duct.

Various nerves are found coursing through the superior mediastinum and, owing to the latter's asymmetry, they have different courses on the two sides. These nerves are the left and right phrenic nerves, the left and right vagus nerves, and the left recurrent laryngeal nerve. Lymph nodes are also to be found in the connective tissue.
[A:1195; C:518; D:44; F:438; G:176]

359 The ligamentum arteriosum is a fibrous band which runs from the commencement of the left

pulmonary artery to the lower concave surface of the aortic arch, and around which the left recurrent laryngeal nerve hooks. It is the remains of the ductus arteriosus of the fetus which conveys blood from the pulmonary trunk to the aorta, bypassing the lungs.

The ductus is derived from the left sixth aortic arch of early embryological development around which the recurrent laryngeal nerve winds, thus accounting for its position in the adult. On the right, the sixth and fifth arches disappear and the nerve is found looping around the fourth arch artery (right subclavian artery of the adult).

[A:158, 616; B:322; D:38; E:84; G:153]

360 The left and right recurrent laryngeal nerves are branches of the left and right vagus nerves, respectively, and their courses are different on the two sides.

The left recurrent laryngeal nerve arises from the left vagus as it crosses the aortic arch. It hooks round the ligamentum arteriosum and ascends on the left in the groove between oesophagus and trachea.

The right recurrent laryngeal nerve arises from the right vagus as it crosses the first part of the subclavian artery. It loops underneath the artery, and ascends on the right between trachea and oesophagus in a similar fashion to the left nerve.

Both nerves pass deep to the lateral lobes of the thyroid gland where they have an intimate relationship with the inferior thyroid artery, passing in front of it or behind it, or through its terminal branches. The nerves pass below the inferior constrictor muscle into the larynx to supply all the laryngeal muscles (except the cricothyroid) and sensation to the mucous membrane below the level of the cords.

[A:158, 1023, 1182; B:333; D:38; F:438; G:963]

D Applied answers

361 The anterior mediastinum is located inferior to the manubriosternal angle, anterior to the pericardium and heart, and posterior to the sternum. Its major component is the thymus gland, which also extends into the superior medias-

tinum. Normally, the thymus is relatively large in children and regresses with age but tumours of this organ may cause obstruction to the many structures passing through the superior mediastinum—in particular the superior vena cava and oesophagus, both of which are compressed relatively easily. A retrosternal goitre may also produce similar symptoms.
[E:100; G:102]

362 The fairly consistent diameters of the trachea and main bronchi are due to the strengthening cartilaginous bands and rings which maintain their shape even during inspiration. The trachea is a membranous tube supported by 15–20 U-shaped bands of hyaline cartilage which are deficient posteriorly. The lowest hyaline band in the trachea is similar in shape to a pair of bathing briefs. The carina separating the main bronchi may be likened to the crutch of the briefs.
[B:281; E:73; G:180; H:185; J:66]

363 The intrinsic muscles of the larynx are all innervated by the recurrent laryngeal nerves save the cricothyroid muscle, which is supplied by the external laryngeal nerve. The origins of these recurrent laryngeal nerves differ—the left leaving the vagus and hooking round the remnant sixth arch, the ductus arteriosus, whilst the right leaves the vagus in the root of the neck and hooks round the right subclavian artery just lateral to the first rib. An apical tumour may therefore readily affect the recurrent laryngeal nerves, especially on the right, by quite minimal local spread.
[E:87; G:180]

364 The lymphatic drainage of the oesophagus is through a plexus of vessels which pass into the posterior mediastinal nodes and along the left gastric vessels through the diaphragm to the coeliac nodes around the aorta. Because of the plexus, however, it is not rare for a lower oesophageal carcinoma to present as hard nodes palpable in the supraclavicular region due to the ascent of lymph into the mediastinum and neck.
[A:747; F:37]

365 Superiorly lies the indentation made by the arch of the aorta; then just inferiorly lies that of the left main bronchus whilst the largest, most inferior, impression is caused by the left atrium.
[I:716; J:234]

366 Vomiting blood (haematemesis) in an alcoholic patient is commonly due to either a peptic ulcer or oesophagogastric varices. These varices are thin-walled, tortuous, dilated veins which lie in the submucosa and lamina propria and are formed at the site of portosystemic venous anastomoses when there is raised portal venous pressure. In this case the cause is likely to be cirrhosis. The submucosal veins receive tributaries from dilated subepithelial veins and drain to the veins found on the oesophageal serosal surface. These veins communicate with both the azygos vein (systemic) and the left gastric veins (portal).
[D:92; E:205; F:217; H:232]

367 Congenital tracheo-oesophageal abnormalities are relatively common quite simply because of the very close developmental origins of the two tubes. The laryngotracheal groove and tube differentiate from the floor of the foregut, so it is not surprising to find the oesophagus ending in a blind pouch whilst there is a fistula between the trachea and lower oesophagus. Sometimes the oesophagus opens into the trachea.
[A:181; D:47]

368 It is most likely to be inhaled into the right main bronchus, which is shorter, wider and nearly in the same direct line as the trachea. The right bronchus is only about 2.5 cm long compared with 5 cm of the left. Once inhaled, material such as peanuts, pins or simply gastric fluid will tend to pass into the right middle or lower lobes. However, in the unconscious patient lying on the right, inhaled material often favours the posterior segment of the upper lobe.
[G:139; H:184; J:66]

ABDOMEN

A   Information answers

369 The abdomen is divided up into nine regions by the construction of two lines in the transverse

plane and two in the sagittal plane, rather as one would construct a frame for a game of noughts and crosses. The upper transverse line is the transpyloric plane at L1/2, which encircles the body at a point half-way between the suprasternal notch and the symphysis pubis. The lower transverse plane is the transtubercular plane at L5, drawn between the two tubercles on the iliac crests. The two vertical lines are the right and left lateral lines. They are constructed by raising perpendiculars to the transverse lines from each mid-inguinal point (half-way between pubic symphysis and anterior superior iliac spine). The median upper portion is termed the epigastric, with a right and left hypochondrial region on either side. The median part of the middle zone is the umbilical, with a right and left lumbar (or lateral) region on either side of it. The median lower portion is termed hypogastric or suprapubic, with a right and left iliac region to each side.
[A:1254; C:559; E:122]

370 The linea alba, linea semilunaris and arcuate lines are all associated with the rectus sheath. The linea alba is a strong fibrous line found in the midline between the two rectus abdominis muscles and formed by the fusion of the aponeuroses of the three abdominal wall muscles. It is attached superiorly to the xiphisternum and inferiorly to the symphysis pubis. The linea semilunaris is formed by the splitting of the aponeurosis of the internal oblique muscle to form the rectus sheath. It marks the lateral border of the rectus sheath and curves (like a half-moon) from the pubic tubercle to the costal margin at the ninth costal cartilage (L1). The internal oblique aponeurosis splits to enclose the rectus sheath, the external oblique passing in front, the transversus behind. At a point just below the umbilicus this arrangement stops. Below this point all the aponeuroses pass anterior to the rectus muscle and the posterior part of the sheath is absent. The posterior sheath thus ends in an abrupt free margin which is convex upwards. This is the arcuate line (Douglas). [A:524; D:61]

371 Above the umbilicus the rectus sheath is arranged as follows. The external oblique aponeu-

rosis passes in front of the muscle, the transversus aponeurosis behind. The aponeurosis of the internal oblique splits to enclose the rectus muscle. At a point just below the umbilicus this arrangement is radically altered. Below this point all the aponeuroses pass anterior to the rectus muscle. The posterior rectus sheath is absent; only transversalis fascia separates the rectus muscle from peritoneum.
[A:524; D:61; E:133; F:178; G:26]

372 The level of L1 is sometimes termed the transpyloric plane (Addison). This transverse plane bisects the body at a level mid-way between the jugular notch and the symphysis pubis. A number of important anatomical structures lie at this level. They are:
   1. Fundus of gall bladder where the plane cuts the right ninth costal cartilage
   2. Pylorus of stomach
   3. Termination of spinal cord
   4. Origin of superior mesenteric artery from aorta
   5. Hila of kidneys and hence renal vessels
   6. Splenic vein and body of pancreas
[D:58; F:191]

373 The sites most commonly affected in herniae are: the region of the inguinal canal (inguinal hernia and femoral hernia), the region of the umbilicus (umbilical hernia) and the rectus sheath (epigastric hernia and Spigelian hernia). For the sake of completeness, lumbar hernia and obturator hernia should be mentioned.
   An inguinal hernia may be indirect or direct. The indirect hernia follows the path taken by the spermatic cord through the deep inguinal ring, along the inguinal canal, exiting through the superficial inguinal ring. It may occur in baby boys, where it is often due to a patent processus vaginalis. The direct inguinal hernia pushes its way into the inguinal canal through a weakened posterior wall. Its origin is therefore medial to the deep inguinal ring. Having entered the canal, it follows the course of the spermatic cord to exit at the superficial inguinal ring.
   A femoral hernia passes through the femoral canal. This is an area of deadspace medial to the femoral vein, containing fat and a lymph node.

Its medial border is the sharp lacunar ligament (on which femoral herniae frequently strangulate). A femoral hernia may easily be distinguished from an inguinal hernia. The latter is palpated at the superficial inguinal ring, which is above and medial to the pubic tubercle. The femoral hernia is below and lateral to the pubic tubercle. An umbilical hernia may be due to congenital failure of contraction of an umbilical scar or due to the umbilical scar giving way in later life.

An epigastric hernia is found above the umbilicus in the midline. It is due to a weakness of the linea alba. A Spigelian hernia is due to a weakness of the arcuate line of the rectus sheath. A lumbar hernia is found in the lumbar triangle behind the free border of the external oblique muscle and above the iliac crest. An obturator hernia passes through the obturator canal where the obturator nerve and vessels run through the membrane covering the obturator foramen. Pressure on the nerve may cause pain in the distribution of the nerve (medial side of thigh and knee). It may appear in the femoral triangle and be confused with the much more common femoral hernia.
[A:1297; D:67; E:160]

374 The superficial fascia of the abdomen is traditionally divided into two: a superficial fatty layer (Camper's fascia) and a deeper membranous layer (Scarpa's fascia). The thickness of the superficial layer varies with the degree of obesity of the individual. There is no deep fascia, otherwise the abdomen could not stretch to accommodate the 'Fs' (food, fluid, faeces, flatus, fetus, intermesenteric fat) with which it may be physiologically or pathologically distended.
[A:519; D:59; E:130; F:175]

375 The conjoint tendon is formed by the fusion of the lowermost and most medial tendinous fibres of the internal oblique and transversus muscles. It is fused medially to the linea alba but has a lateral free border. Inferiorly it is attached to the pecten of the pubis. The conjoint tendon is situated behind the superficial inguinal ring. It provides some posterior support to this weak area of the abdominal wall.
[A:523; E:135; F:180; G:211]

376   The testis is covered by a thick indistensible covering of fibrous tissue called the tunica albuginea. Each of the three erectile portions of the penis is covered by a tough fibrous fascia also termed the tunica albuginea. In the female the ovary possesses a tunica albuginea. It is a delicate layer of fibrous tissue situated immediately beneath the germinal epithelium.
[A:1337, 1347, 1352; B:468; E:142; F:186]

377   The vas deferens (ductus deferens) is easily palpated within the spermatic cord. It is supplied with blood from its own private artery, the artery to the vas deferens. This arises from either the superior vesical artery or the inferior vesical artery, both of which are branches of the internal iliac artery.
[A:1343; B:468; D:67; E:142; G:220]

378   The spermatozoa commence their journey at their site of production—the seminiferous tubules of the testis. These drain into the mediastinum of the testis where a network of anastomosing tubules is situated, the rete testis. From the rete testis the spermatozoa pass along some six to twelve efferent ductules into the head of the epididymis. Here the ductules coalesce to form a single duct of the epididymis. This much-coiled tube is situated in the body and tail of the structure. From the tail of the epididymis the spermatozoa drain into the vas deferens (ductus deferens). This is the continuation of the duct of the epididymis and traverses the scrotum and inguinal canal. At the deep ring, it hooks round the lateral side of the inferior epigastric vessels and runs subperitoneally around the pelvic wall to the base of the bladder, looping anterior to the ureter as it does so. The distal portion of the vas is dilated as the ampulla. The terminal end joins the duct of the seminal vesicle on the bladder base to form the ejaculatory duct, which pierces the prostate gland to enter the urethra at the side of the urethral crest.
[A:1336–44; B:469; F:225; G:217]

379   The superficial fascia of the scrotum is entirely devoid of fat. It contains the dartos muscle, which is a thin layer of unstriped fibres supplied by autonomic nerves.
[A:1345; B:501; D:126; E:145]

380 In the male the paramesonephric ducts (Müllerian ducts) disappear except at their upper and lower ends. The upper end forms the appendix testis in the adult male, the lower end forms the utriculus masculinus in the prostate. Note that descent of the testes into the scrotum reverses the relationships of these structures in the adult with respect to the embryo.
[A:187; F:187]

A Applied answers

381 The skin of the anterior abdominal wall is divided into rough quadrants with respect to its lymphatic drainage. There is a fairly constant watershed at the level of the umbilicus as if a belt were fastened here. Above the belt the lymphatic drainage of the skin goes to the anterior axillary or pectoral lymph nodes while below it goes to the superficial inguinal nodes, and thus all quadrants will be affected in paraumbilical tattoo.
[A:741; F:176]

382 An indirect inguinal hernia passes through the deep or internal ring lateral to the inferior epigastric vessels and along the canal. Sometimes, if large enough, it may pass into the scrotum after emerging through the superficial inguinal ring. A direct inguinal hernia passes anteriorly through the posterior wall of the inguinal canal and lies medial to the inferior epigastric vessels. It normally passes through a naturally weak region in the inferior portion of the inguinal triangle (Hesselbach) and, due to the presence of the strong conjoint tendon far medially, often has a wide neck. Clinical examination, however, is poor for distinguishing these two prior to operation.

Baby boys tend to present with indirect herniae because this is the same path that the gubernaculum and processus vaginalis take during development. Persistence of the processus as a small sac may result in an indirect hernia, especially following increased intra-abdominal pressure when abdominal contents may be forced into this waiting peritoneal recess.
[A:1297; D:67; E:161]

383 McBurney's point is two-thirds of the way along a line from the umbilicus to the right anterior superior iliac spine. It is a landmark for a classic gridiron incision used during appendicectomy.
[B:392; H:206]

384 A gridiron incision (also known as muscle-splitting or McBurney's incision) is performed for appendicectomy. The beauty is that each layer of muscle can be retracted and split in the direction of its fibres and thus no cutting is required. Because each muscle layer is directioned differently, when finished this operation wound is very well protected and reinforced, rarely resulting in incisional herniae. The external oblique muscle fibres and aponeurosis run inferiorly and medially, internal oblique fibres run superiorly and medially, and the transversus fibres lie, as their name suggests, transversely.
[D:64; E:160]

385 Abdominal paracentesis is performed through various sites, the most popular being either the avascular linea alba, one-third of the way along a line from the umbilicus to the pubic symphysis, or over the iliac fossae lateral to the linea semilunaris. In the midline the trocar pierces in succession the skin, superficial fasciae and the tough linea alba. It then passes through the transversalis fascia, extraperitoneal fat and the parietal peritoneum before entering the peritoneal cavity. In using a more lateral approach, the three flat abdominal muscles—external oblique, internal oblique and the transversus abdominis—are pierced prior to the transversalis fascia. It is normal clinical practice to empty the bladder prior to paracentesis to avoid its being punctured!
[A:524; D:65; E:164]

386 The segmental nerve supply to rectus abdominis is from the lower thoracic spinal nerves, which enter the muscle along its lateral border. During paramedian incisions the rectus muscle should therefore be retracted laterally to avoid trauma to these segmental nerves.
[D:63; E:159; G:28]

387 The Pfannenstiel incision is a transverse suprapubic incision performed for pelvic surgery.
Depending on how far laterally it is extended, it
involves the rectus sheath and muscles in the
midline as well as the oblique and transverse
abdominal muscles laterally. Due to the lateral
innervation, it is rare to damage more than one
segmental nerve, thus providing a strong postoperative scar. The closure is made in layers
and, provided the anterior rectus sheath is well
sutured, it is unnecessary to suture the muscle
itself. The posterior rectus sheath at this level is
almost non-existent, as the aponeuroses of the
flat abdominal muscles lie anterior to rectus
abdominis.
[A:526; C:566]

388 Collateral vessels available in cases of inferior
vena caval block include the superficial and
inferior epigastric veins, which carry the blood
to the thoracoepigastric and superior epigastric
veins and hence to the lateral veins and into the
superior vena cava. Clinically, this passage of
blood may be seen and felt as a tortuous vari-
cosed large vein from groin to axilla. Other
smaller channels occur between the pelvic
veins, vertebral venous system and superior
vena cava, as well as the azygos system.
[A:709; F:477]

389 If your patient was unlucky enough to have his
ilioinguinal nerve trapped in the hernia repair,
pain may be felt in the L1 dermatome, which
includes the scrotum.
[A:1051; G:211]

390 The testis is an internal organ and so the pain is
felt as referred pain. Trauma to the testes is felt
as a non-specific paraumbilical pain due to the
testes' T10 innervation. Remember that it descends from the posterior abdominal wall. The
T10 dermatome is in the region of the umbilicus.
[A:1343; C:642]

391 The lymphatic drainage of the scrotum is similar to all that of the skin below the umbilicus
and goes therefore to the superficial inguinal
nodes. The testis, however, is an abdominal
organ which descends during development

from the posterior abdominal wall through the inguinal canal and into the scrotum. It brings its vascular supply from the abdominal aorta and its lymphatics drain to the para-aortic nodes situated just below the level of the renal veins. This difference in lymphatic spread may have serious consequences in patients with testicular tumours.

[A:734, 741; C:736]

392 A hydrocele is an abnormal collection of fluid between the parietal and visceral layers of the tunica vaginalis of the testis. It could be compared to a pleural effusion or ascites. Aspiration of this fluid with trocar and cannula is rarely of permanent relief, as the cause of increased serous fluid production has not been removed. It is therefore sometimes necessary surgically to obliterate the cavity of the tunica vaginalis to cure a hydrocele. A varicocele is a swelling of the pampiniform plexus of veins draining the epididymis and testis. It is seen more commonly on the left side and may be described by the patient as 'varicose veins in the scrotum'.

[D:129; E:168]

393 A vasectomy is usually performed in the upper part of the scrotum just before the spermatic cord enters the superficial inguinal ring. To reach the vas, the three major coverings will have to be incised, viz. the external spermatic fascia derived from the external oblique aponeurosis, the cremasteric fascia and muscle derived from the internal oblique muscle and the internal spermatic fascia from the transversalis fascia. The easily palpable vas will now lie exposed and surrounded by numerous vessels and lymphatics.

[A:1343; G:221]

394 The gubernaculum ovarii becomes both the ligament of the ovary and the round ligament of the uterus in the adult female. They are usually continuous and attach to the uterus just below the uterine tube. The round ligament takes a course very similar to the male ductus deferens, passing along the inguinal canal and ending in the female scrotal homologue, the labium majus.

[A:190; C:692; E:144]

B   Information answers

395   The stomach is found in the epigastrium and left hypochondrium, the spleen in the left hypochondrium. The bulk of the liver is in the right hypochondrium but it extends into the epigastrium and the left hypochondrium. The ileocaecal valve is in the right iliac region.
[A:1254; D:58; E:125; H:206]

396   The spleen, liver and transverse colon are covered in peritoneum and are suspended from the abdominal wall by mesenteries. They are intraperitoneal. The kidney is developed in the posterior abdominal wall behind the peritoneal cavity. Certain parts of the kidneys just happen to have peritoneum on their anterior aspect. They are extraperitoneal. The pancreas and duodenum are peculiar. As gut structures they originally developed intraperitoneally with mesenteries. However, these have become absorbed to leave the pancreas and duodenum stuck on the posterior abdominal wall covered with peritoneum only on their anterior aspect. These organs are described therefore as extraperitoneal, and, save for the first few centimetres, the duodenum is not easily movable.
[A:1262; B:369; C:116, 586]

397   A mesentery is any double-layered fold of peritoneum which attaches intestine to the abdominal wall. It provides the means whereby blood vessels, lymphatics and nerves supply the relevant portion of the intestine. THE mesentery is a mesentery which attaches the jejunum and ileum to the posterior abdominal wall. It extends from the duodenojejunal junction (at the left side of L2), downwards and to the right for 15 cm, to terminate at the ileocaecal junction (over the right sacroiliac joint).
[A:1266; B:368]

398   The epiploic foramen (Winslow) leads from the greater sac of the peritoneum into the lesser sac. The foramen admits two fingers and its boundaries are:
   anteriorly the free border of the lesser omentum with the three structures contained therein (hepatic artery, hepatic portal vein, common bile duct)
   posteriorly the inferior vena cava

173

superiorly the caudate process of the liver
inferiorly the first part of the duodenum.

Sometimes bowel herniates through the foramen and becomes incarcerated or strangulated. In these circumstances, decompression is difficult because all the boundaries of the foramen are vital structures and cannot be incised.
[A:1262; F:198]

399 The epiploic foramen leads from the greater sac into the right of the lesser sac (omental bursa). This pouch of the peritoneal cavity is found posterior to the stomach and lesser omentum. It extends inferiorly between the leaves of the greater omentum and superiorly between liver anteriorly, diaphragm posteriorly, inferior vena cava to the right and oesophagus to the left (upper recess). Its left limit is formed by the spleen. It provides a bursa on which the stomach may slide across the structures of the posterior abdominal wall.
[A:1263; E:180; F:198]

400 In development, the foregut has two mesenteries—ventral and dorsal. The remainder of the gut has only a dorsal mesentery. Thus the ventral foregut mesentery has a free inferior border which extends from the umbilicus to the foregut–midgut junction. The liver develops in this ventral mesentery dividing it into two: the falciform ligament from anterior abdominal wall to liver, and lesser omentum from liver to gut. In the adult, therefore, the falciform ligament is a sickle-shaped double-layered fold of peritoneum. It extends in a line from the diaphragm and anterior abdominal wall as far inferiorly as the umbilicus. It runs onto the liver round which it then splits to enclose. It has a free lower edge in which is situated the ligamentum teres—the remains of the left umbilical vein.
[A:1303; B:373; E:178; G:227]

401 The greater omentum is the mesentery which attaches the stomach to the posterior abdominal wall. Like any other mesentery, it consists of two layers of peritoneum with blood vessels, nerves, lymphatics and fat between the layers. However, the greater omentum is much too big merely to pass straight back from stomach to

174

posterior abdominal wall, and instead it hangs down in front of the intestines like an apron. A transverse section in this area would cut through peritoneum four times, once through the double-layered anterior leaf and once through the double-layered posterior leaf. Between the anterior and posterior leaves is the lesser sac. It should be said that the two double-layered leaves of peritoneum frequently become fused, obliterating the space between them. Similarly, the transverse mesocolon becomes adherent to the posterior aspect of the greater omentum.
[A:1265; B:371; D:69]

402 The lesser omentum is a double-layered mesentery of peritoneum. It stretches in a line from the right side of the abdominal oesophagus, the lesser curve of the stomach and first 2 cm of the first part of the duodenum to the undersurface of the liver. The lesser omentum ends in a right free border, extending from the first part of the duodenum to the porta hepatis. In the free border are contained three vital structures: the hepatic portal vein posteriorly, the common bile duct anteriorly and on the right, and the hepatic artery anteriorly and on the left.
[A:1265; C:371; D:69; F:194]

403 The liver is not wholly covered by peritoneum but has a bare area posteriorly. At the bare area the liver and diaphragm are in direct apposition. The reflections of peritoneum from diaphragm to liver at the margins of the bare area constitute the coronary ligament. It has two leaves—an upper and a lower, at respective limits of the bare area. At the left and right margins of the bare area the leaves of the coronary ligament run for a short while in apposition before becoming continuous. These constitute the right and left triangular ligaments.
[A:1258; E:211; F:200]

404 The lienorenal ligament is part of the dorsal mesentery of the foregut. It extends from the region of the left kidney as a two-layered fold of peritoneum to the spleen. It forms the left margin of the omental bursa. Between its leaves

are the tail of the pancreas and the splenic vessels.
[A:1262; D:69; E:179]

405 Normal females have two openings into their peritoneal cavity at the ovarian end of the Fallopian tubes. This communication (between peritoneal cavity and the exterior) may be readily visualised radiographically in a hystero-salpingogram. Contrast medium is introduced through the cervix, into the uterine cavity and along the tubes. A free spill of medium into the peritoneal cavity demonstrates the patency of the tubes. This route, from the exterior to peritoneal cavity, may be followed by infection and is a documented, though rare, cause of peritonitis.
[A:1356; J:206]

406 The median umbilical ligament is the fibrous remnant of the urachus. It is a midline fibrous cord joining the apex of the bladder to the umbilicus. The urachus originally joined the embryonic cloaca with the allantois in the umbilical cord. Sometimes it remains patent and a newborn baby is found to have urine dribbling from its umbilicus. The medial umbilical ligaments are the fibrous remnants of the umbilical arteries of the fetus, originally branches of the internal iliac artery.
[A:1258; F:204]

B Applied answers

407 Definite structures that form within the ventral mesentery or septum include the falciform ligament, liver and gall bladder and the lesser omentum. The other interesting structure from this region is the ventral part of the pancreas, which is an outgrowth from the primitive bile duct. It eventually becomes the lower part of the head of the pancreas and the proximal portion of the main pancreatic duct (Wirsung). This development explains the common openings of the pancreatic and biliary ducts at the duodenal ampulla (Vater). The ventral mesentery has a free caudal edge which becomes the anterior border of the epiploic foramen.
[A:178; E:216]

408 Ascites is an abnormal collection of fluid within the peritoneal cavity. It therefore lies between the parietal and visceral layers of peritoneum and is a similar situation to a hydrocele or a pleural or pericardial effusion, each within their serous sacs.
[A:1257; E:164]

409 The structures posterior to the lesser sac form the classic 'stomach bed' and include the diaphragm, pancreas, left kidney and suprarenal gland. Other structures include the transverse mesocolon, duodenum, spleen and its vessels.
[E:188; G:274]

410 The epiploic foramen is the opening into the lesser sac and marks the right or free edge of the lesser omentum. This contains the hepatic artery, bile ducts and portal vein and the cystic artery, which arises from the right hepatic artery though it is prone to anomalies. Thus a bleeding gall bladder operation may be assisted by simple two-finger pressure on the hepatic artery lying in the free edge of the lesser omentum just anterior to the foramen.
[A:1265; G:228, 232]

411 For a volvulus to occur there must be a certain freedom of movement of the bowel concerned. The descending colon rarely has any mesentery worth discussing, whilst the sigmoid colon normally has a quite respectable mesocolon which, if too long and mobile, is likely to twist on itself. Interestingly, this condition of sigmoid volvulus is quite common in African races who have a high fibre diet and relatively long sigmoid colons.
[A:1296; B:371]

412 The appendix is a viscera, so early inflammation is evident as referred pain to the small gut dermatome of T10 (i.e. the region of the umbilicus). When, however, the local parietal—as distinct from visceral—peritoneum is involved, the pain is experienced at the site of inflammation, usually in the right iliac fossa near the classic site of McBurney's point.
[C:642; H:206]

413 The subphrenic spaces are potential spaces within the peritoneal cavity, which may become filled with pus and form subphrenic abscesses. The right and left subphrenic spaces lie between the diaphragm and the liver but are separated from each other by the falciform ligament. Both spaces have as their anterior boundary the abdominal wall and their superior limit the diaphragm. The posterior border on the right is the coronary ligament and on the left the left triangular ligament. Clinically, the right space is the more important.
[A:1262; E:185]

C Information answers

414 During their thoracic course, the vagi eventually come to lie on the oesophagus—the right vagus on its right and left vagus on the left. These nerves then divide up to form the oesophageal plexus. At the lower extremity of the oesophagus the vagi become reconstituted. However, owing to the rotation of the stomach during development, the reconstituted vagi lie not left and right but are situated anteriorly and posteriorly as the anterior and posterior vagal trunks, respectively. In this position they pierce the diaphragm with the oesophagus and enter the abdomen.
[A:1021; F:219; G:162]

415 The stomach is innervated by autonomic nerves of the sympathetic and parasympathetic systems.

The sympathetic nerves are derived from segments T6, 7, 8 and 9. Their preganglionic fibres pass through the diaphragm as the splanchnic nerves and relay in the coeliac ganglia to be distributed to the stomach via blood vessels.

The parasympathetic fibres are derived from the vagal trunks. Both vagal trunks run on their respective aspects of the lesser curvature and send branches to the anterior and posterior surfaces of the stomach. The anterior vagal trunk also sends branches to the liver via the lesser omentum. Recurrent branches from here sweep back to supply the pyloric region.
[A:1275; D:76; E:191]

416 The stomach bed is composed of those structures which lie behind the stomach and are separated from it by the lesser sac (omental bursa). These structures are the diaphragm, left suprarenal gland (and upper part of left kidney), the pancreas, spleen, splenic vessels and the transverse mesocolon.
[A:1271; E:188; G:274]

417 The artery of the foregut and foregut derivatives is the coeliac axis (trunk). The foregut extends as far inferiorly as the entry of the bile duct into the second part of the duodenum and consists of the lower oesophagus, stomach and the proximal duodenum, liver, spleen and proximal part of the pancreas.
[A:174; E:204; G:244]

418 The lymphatic drainage of the stomach closely follows its arterial supply and the nodes can therefore be conveniently divided into four groups. The lymph nodes around the left gastric vessels receive lymph from the left half of the lesser curvature. From this group, efferents pass to the coeliac nodes around the coeliac artery. The lymph nodes around the right gastric vessels receive lymph from the right half of the lesser curvature. From here, efferents pass along the hepatic artery and to the coeliac nodes. The left portion of the greater curvature sends its lymph along the short gastric and left gastroepiploic arteries to nodes in the hilum of the spleen. From here, efferents pass to the pancreaticosplenic nodes along the course of the splenic artery to the coeliac nodes. Lymph from the right portion of the greater curve follows the gastroepiploic artery, which has nodes along its length. Efferents follow the gastroduodenal artery to the coeliac nodes.
[A:738; E:191]

419 The small intestine changes its character gradually throughout its length, jejenum merging imperceptibly into ileum. However, various features distinguish proximal jejunum from terminal ileum. The jejunum has a thicker wall owing to the thicker and more numerous mucosal folds (valvulae conniventes) in this region. The mesentery has more fat between its layers in the ileum as compared with the jejunum. In

the latter it is relatively transparent, forming 'windows' between the blood vessels. In the former, the fat makes it opaque. The mesenteric blood vessels form only one or two (anastomosing) loops or arcades to the jejunum. The ileum possesses up to half a dozen shorter layers of arcades. The jejunum is of greater diameter than the ileum. Furthermore, the ileum contains aggregations of lymphoid tissue (Peyer's patches) which are absent from the jejunum.
[A:1279; D:80; E:197]

420 The autonomic supply to the intestine may be divided into two: the sympathetic and the parasympathetic innervation.

The sympathetic innervation is derived from the thoracic sympathetic trunk as the splanchnic nerves. These contain preganglionic fibres and pierce the diaphragm to synapse in the coeliac plexuses situated on each side of the coeliac artery.

The parasympathetic supply is derived from the vagus. A large branch passes from the posterior vagal trunk in company with the left gastric artery, to the coeliac plexus. The parasympathetic fibres eventually synapse in their target organs, the postganglionic fibres being extremely short. From the coeliac plexus, branches of both sympathetic and parasympathetic systems pass with the coeliac and superior mesenteric arteries to the intestine.
[A:1077; E:230]

421 The large bowel is usually of larger calibre than the small intestine. Its mucosa is featureless whereas the small intestine is folded and feels velvety, owing to villi. The colon carries fat-filled tags in its peritoneal covering—the appendices epiploicae. These are absent in the small intestine. The outer longitudinal muscle coat of the large intestine is not as complete as that of the small intestine. Instead it is condensed into three flattened bands, called taeniae coli, set at regular intervals around the circumference of the bowel. These taeniae are shorter than the rest of the large bowel and therefore throw it into characteristic sacculations. In contrast, the small bowel is of uniform width with no sacculations.
[A:1284; D:81]

422   The junction between the midgut and the hind-gut is situated between the right two-thirds and left third of the transverse colon. The midgut portion is supplied by the superior mesenteric artery via the middle colic branch, the hindgut portion is supplied by the inferior mesenteric artery via the left colic branch. These arteries anastomose along the mesenteric border of the colon by means of the marginal artery (Drum-mond).
[A:664; F:225; G:250]

423   The pelvic mesocolon is a mesentery which attaches the sigmoid colon to the posterior pelvic wall. It has the shape of an inverted V. The apex is situated at the point of division of the left common iliac artery. The left ureter runs behind it. The right limb passes downwards and to the right and ends in the midline at the level of the third sacral vertebra. The left limb descends on the medial side of the left psoas muscle.
[A:1266; B:370]

C Applied answers

424   Congenital hypertrophic pyloric stenosis is a thickening of the pyloric sphincter, found more commonly in first-born male children, which interferes with normal gastric emptying. Classi-cally, it presents with the advent of projectile vomiting when the child is about 6 weeks old. It is cured by simple splitting of the hypertrophic muscle; it has been noted that the intramural ganglia cells are reduced in this region, though the aetiology of the disease is not fully under-stood.
[A:1273; C:606]

425   Vagotomy is performed to reduce the gastric secretion, most commonly in cases of peptic ulceration. The anterior and posterior vagal trunks enter the abdomen through the oeso-phageal hiatus in the right crus of the dia-phragm. The surgeon who wishes to perform total or truncal vagotomy will find the oesopha-gus the most useful landmark. The anterior vagus lies very close to the stomach and sup-plies the cardia, lesser curvature, liver and a

clinically important branch to the upper border of pylorus and antrum (nerve of Latarjet). The posterior vagal trunk supplies the body of the stomach but its largest branch is via the coeliac ganglion to the rest of the fore- and midgut. As the vagus is both motor and secretory to the stomach, it is often necessary to combine vagotomy with a drainage procedure such as widening the pylorus (pyloroplasty). Due to its far-reaching innervation (L. *vagus* = a wanderer), a vagotomy is occasionally accompanied by severe gastrointestinal upset, most commonly seen as severe diarrhoea.
[D:76; E:192]

426   Occasionally, direct involvement of the pancreas—which is a posterior relation of the stomach and part of its 'bed'—may block the pancreatic ducts. More commonly, pancreatic problems are due to indirect lymph node involvement. The inferior part of the greater curvature of the stomach drains along the right gastroepiploic vessels to the subpyloric group which lies in the head of the pancreas. It is via these nodes that the pancreas may be involved.
[A:738; E:188; G:274]

427   The greater omentum is the 'policeman of the abdomen', as it looks for trouble and then cordons it off. This can readily be seen when opening up the peritoneal cavity in acute appendicitis, when the first structure to pop into view is often the greater omentum trying to seal off the potentially dangerous culprit.
[A:1265; B:371; E:249]

428   Following rupture of the bowel, gas may escape into the cavity. Clinically, this is most commonly seen in perforated peptic ulcer. A common cause nowadays for gas being in the cavity is following gas insufflation, mainly carbon dioxide, as used in laparoscopy, peritoneoscopy, hysterosalpingography or other x-ray procedures. It is demonstrated radiologically by seeing a thin gas shadow between the liver and diaphragm on a plain erect abdominal x-ray. This must not be confused with a normal stomach gas bubble.
[E:185; J:58]

429 The rule of twos: Meckel's diverticulum is 2 inches long, seen twice as often in male as female, occurs from 2 feet to 2 metres from the ileocaecal valve along the antimesenteric border of the ileum and occurs in 2 per cent of the population. It is, in fact, the remnant of the vitellointestinal duct. (With apologies to the metric system!)
[B:375; C:597; D:97]

430 Remnants of the vitellointestinal duct vary from a Meckel's diverticulum or a cord which attaches the ileum to the umbilicus, to a 'raspberry' tumour at the umbilicus due to diverticular mucosa. The diverticulum itself may contain gastric or pancreatic mucosa which can lead to ulceration and perforation, clinically mimicking appendicitis. Bowel obstruction can occur as it loops round a remnant cord but potentially more dangerous is using this ileal cord as an axis of rotation which may result in a complete volvulus of the ileum.
[A:1280; D:98; E:158]

431 On barium x-rays, the small bowel is seen centrally placed with plicae circulares (valvulae conniventes), commencing in the second part of the duodenum but disappearing about mid-ileum. These are especially well seen on a small bowel enema, double air contrast x-ray. Because of this feature, the bowel has a 'feather-painted' appearance of barium. The large bowel, however, is positioned more peripherally, the caecum, hepatic flexure and splenic flexure being obvious landmarks. On a standard barium enema sacculations can be seen especially in the transverse colon but this normal haustral pattern is best demonstrated by double air contrast x-rays. This pattern is due to the relative shortness of the longitudinal muscle of the colon, forming three bands of taeniae coli, compared to that of the circular muscle fibres. This results in a bunching up of the bowel wall into sacculations rather like material where a thread has accidentally been pulled.
[J:244, 248]

432 Occasionally during fetal life the caecum will adhere to the visceral liver surface; more commonly however, following rotation of the mid-

gut and its return to the peritoneal cavity, the ascending colon fails to develop, leaving the caecum in the right hypochondrium. This may result in appendicitis being mistaken for cholecystitis.
[A:173; C:375]

433 The region of the large bowel around the splenic flexure is occasionally involved in ischaemic problems, as it is here that the middle colic artery of the superior mesenteric and the upper left colic artery of the inferior mesenteric artery both anastomose. This region of the bowel is therefore supplied only by small terminal branches of the above and the very thin marginal artery (Drummond) which is easily blocked by atheroma.
[A:665; C:601]

434 The sites of diverticulosis, or herniation of the mucosa through the muscle wall, are where the bowel wall is weakest. These sites are between the taeniae coli where there is only circular muscle fibres and particularly where the blood vessels pierce these fibres.
[E:253]

D   Information answers

435 The pancreas is derived from two buds—a dorsal and a ventral—which develop in the respective foregut omenta. The dorsal bud forms the head, body and tail of the adult pancreas; the ventral bud forms the uncinate process. During development the ventral bud somehow revolves round the circumference of the duodenum, passing behind it, to lie in line with and underneath the dorsal bud. The superior mesenteric vessels pass below this dorsal bud. Migration of the ventral bud behind the duodenum causes the ventral bud to lie behind the superior mesenteric vessels. In the adult pancreas the superior mesenteric vessels are therefore seen to pass between the dorsal and ventral buds (i.e. between the body and the uncinate process). It therefore appears as if the pancreas has been pierced by these vessels.
[A:179, 1300; F:227; G:285]

436 The pancreas lies on the posterior abdominal wall behind the lesser sac. The tail of the pancreas, however, turns forwards in the lieno-renal ligament and usually lies in contact with the gastric impression of the spleen. It may be damaged during splenectomy.
[A:1299; F:233]

437 The duodenum is some 25 cm long and is a C-shaped tube concave to the left. The head of the pancreas lies within this concavity. The duodenum is divided into four parts. The first part commences at the pylorus at the level of L1, 2 cm to the right of the midline, and runs upwards, backwards and to the right, anterior to and across the right side of L1. The second part of the duodenum runs vertically downwards on the right side of the vertebral column from L1 to L3. The third part runs horizontally to the left, anterior to and across the body of L3. The fourth part runs upwards and to the left, eventually to turn forwards at the level of L1, 2 cm to the left of the midline as the duodeno-jejunal junction.
[A:1277; H:203; J:236]

438 Being a gut derivative, the venous drainage of the spleen must be to the portal system. The splenic vein commences by the joining of some half dozen splenic tributaries which leave the spleen at the hilum. The single vessel runs in the lienorenal ligament to the posterior abdominal wall, where it runs downwards and to the right.

It is situated at a lower level than the artery and therefore runs behind the body of the pancreas where it receives the inferior mesenteric vein. It is not tortuous, unlike the artery. It ends behind the neck of the pancreas, where it joins the superior mesenteric vein to form the portal vein.
[A:710; E:205]

439 The spleen originally develops as separate discrete masses of splenic tissue, called splenunculi, in the dorsal mesentery of the foregut. Each splenunculus has its own artery and vein. During development, the splenunculi fuse to form the definitive spleen. However, incomplete fusion at the anterior margin results in the characteristic notches. Sometimes fusion of the

splenunculi is even less complete, resulting in accessory spleens. The typical division of the splenic vessels as they enter the spleen is due to the fact that the terminal vessels supply the remains of one splenunculus apiece. They are end vessels, with no anastomoses. This explains the predilection of the spleen to suffer typical wedge-shaped infarcts if any of these terminal branches is occluded.
[A:180; H:233]

440 The spleen is ovoid in shape with a convex diaphragmatic surface and a concave visceral surface, which contains the hilum centrally and has further concave impressions for stomach, colon and left kidney. The vessels enter and leave at the hilum. Its anterior border is characteristically notched. Its long axis lies along the left tenth rib, the spleen extending between the ninth and eleventh ribs. It extends usually no further anteriorly than the mid-axillary line. The numbers 1, 3, 5, 7, 9 and 11 summarise some important facts concerning the spleen. It measures $1 \times 3 \times 5$ inches, weighs 7 oz. and lies between the ninth and eleventh ribs. This information does not yield itself easily to metric conversion!
[A:721; D:58; E:218]

441 Being a foregut derivative, the spleen must derive its blood supply from the foregut artery (coeliac artery). Thus the splenic artery arises from the coeliac artery and passes to the left behind the posterior peritoneal wall of the lesser sac. It is noted for its remarkable tortuosity and this causes it to alternately appear and disappear behind the upper border of the pancreas in this region. It crosses anterior to the left suprarenal gland and upper part of the left kidney and enters the lienorenal ligament to reach the spleen. On its arrival it divides into several terminal branches which enter the hilum. It supplies the pancreas as it passes along it via small pancreatic branches, and also the stomach via the left gastroepiploic artery (which arises near its termination and runs in the gastrosplenic ligament) and the short gastric arteries.
[A:661; F:214]

D Applied answers

442 The pancreas develops from two separate regions. The greater part of the pancreas originates in the dorsal mesentery and this forms the body and tail. The spleen also develops within this mesentery, thus helping one to remember the close relationship of the tail of the pancreas with the hilum of the spleen. The head of the pancreas, however, develops in the ventral mesentery from the bile duct bud. Later, during gut rotation, the ventral pancreas rotates posterior to the duodenum to form part of the head and uncinate process of the pancreas. The terminal part of the accessory duct normally degenerates, whilst the distal portion of this duct fuses with the short ventral duct to become the main pancreatic duct of Wirsung. This explains how the two parts of the pancreas squeeze the origin of the superior mesenteric vessels like a clothes peg to hold it in line.
[A:179; D:109; F:227]

443 The biliary duct system is best seen by either an intravenous cholangiogram or per- or postoperative cholangiograms when water-soluble contrast medium is injected via the bile ducts through a tube left in situ during cholecystectomy. More recently, a percutaneous transhepatic cholangiogram has gained favour but this involves piercing the liver substance with a fine needle, and therefore presents more potential problems. An oral cholecystogram, though excellent for demonstrating the gall bladder, rarely shows the duct system. The pancreatic ducts can now be outlined radiologically, the most popular approach being a retrograde one with aid of an endoscope under direct vision. This is called an endoscopic retrograde cholangiopancreatogram (ERCP). Quite often the distal pancreatic duct may be seen on a cholangiogram due to reflux from the duodenal ampulla.
[J:250–257]

444 The main pancreatic duct of Wirsung and the common bile duct have a common final pathway and sphincter at the hepatopancreatic ampulla (Vater). Hence a cancer in the head of the pancreas may not only block pancreatic outflow but also commonly presents as obstructive

jaundice by blocking the distal portion of the common bile duct.
[D:107; E:215]

445 A tumour in the posterior part of the neck and head of the pancreas can easily press on the inferior vena cava and cause obstruction to the venous return from the lower limbs.
[A:1299; F:227; G:285]

446 A ruptured spleen will cause an intraperitoneal collection of blood which will tend to gravitate towards the pelvic cavity or subphrenic spaces in the supine position. In this case, the left cupola (dome) of the diaphragm is irritated by a fluid collection in the left subphrenic space. This irritation is felt as referred pain from the diaphragm, whose nerve supply is the phrenic nerve. The phrenic nerve consists of C3, 4 and 5 fibres and the pain is thus referred to the C4 dermatome on the shoulder.
[A:723; B:404; E:207]

447 The duodenum is a C-shaped section of bowel enclosing the head of the pancreas. As it leaves the pylorus, the first few centimetres are covered with peritoneum. However, for the remaining 20 cm, it is a retroperitoneal organ, making mobilisation difficult.
[A:1262; C:582]

E Information answers

448 The lobes of the liver are right, left, quadrate and caudate. The right and left lobes are separated by the attachment of the falciform ligament. The caudate and quadrate lobes are situated on the inferior (visceral) aspects. The quadrate lobe is situated anteriorly between the ligamentum teres, porta hepatis and gall bladder. The caudate lobe is situated posteriorly between the groove for the ligamentum venosum, the inferior vena cava and the porta hepatis. These lobes are demarcated by the attachment of peritoneum and are not functionally distinct. The quadrate and caudate lobes are functionally part of the left lobe and are supplied by the left branches of hepatic

artery and portal vein, and are drained by the left hepatic duct.
[A:1304; D:101]

449   The blood vessels supplying the liver are the hepatic artery and the portal vein. The hepatic artery is a branch of the coeliac axis, the foregut artery. This is logical, as the liver is derived from the foregut region. The hepatic artery supplies oxygenated arterial blood. The portal vein conveys blood to the liver from the gut (and gut derivatives). It is venous and rich in substances absorbed from the bowel. Both the hepatic artery and the portal vein reach the liver by ascending in the free edge of the lesser omentum. When they reach the liver they divide into right and left branches supplying each functional lobe. The liver is drained by hepatic veins. They are usually three in number (left, right and central) and they drain directly into the inferior vena cava as it passes through the liver.
[A:1306; D:101; F:215]

450   The bare area of the liver is situated on the posterior aspect of the right lobe. It is so named because it is devoid of peritoneal covering, unlike the rest of the liver. The bare area is triangular in shape—base to the left, apex to the right. The apex is the right triangular ligament. The sides are the widely separated leaves of the coronary ligament. The base is the left margin of the inferior vena cava.
[A:1258; F:200]

451   The surface marking of the liver may be projected on the body wall as follows. The upper border is a horizontal line passing just below each nipple. The lower border is an oblique line running from the tip of the right tenth rib to the left nipple. Thus the bulk of the liver lies under the rib cage but is uncovered in the epigastrium. In a thin individual it may therefore be palpated, especially in deep inspiration, particularly if it is firmer than usual.
[A:1302; D:58; E:125]

452   In the fetus, oxygenated blood full of nutrients returns from the placenta in the cord via the umbilical vein. The umbilical vein enters the

umbilicus and runs in the free edge of the falciform ligament to the liver. Here it joins the left branch of the portal vein to form the ductus venosus. Some blood passes to the liver, but most bypasses it and runs to the inferior vena cava in the ductus venosus. (It is not necessary for the fetal liver to detoxify the nutrients in this blood, as this has already been done by the maternal liver.)

After birth, the cord is ligated and blood ceases to flow in the umbilical vein. Without the large quantity of blood flowing through it, the ductus venosus collapses. Eventually the ductus venosus and umbilical vein are obliterated and form fibrous cords—the ligamentum venosum and the ligamentum teres respectively.
[A:613; B:320; G:220]

453 The porta hepatis is where the blood vessels and ducts enter and leave the liver. It is situated on the inferior aspect of the organ. The upper extremity of the free edge of the lesser omentum is attached around it. The ducts and vessels bifurcate prior to their entry into the liver, so right and left branches of the hepatic artery and portal vein and right and left hepatic ducts are situated here. Autonomic nerves enter the liver at the porta hepatis, and lymph vessels emerge. Some lymph nodes are situated in this region.
[A:1305; B:396; G:254]

454 The right and left hepatic ducts emerge from their respective lobes of the liver and unite to form a common hepatic duct. The common hepatic duct is some 3.5 cm long. It descends in the free edge of the lesser omentum. A diverticulum—the cystic duct—leaves its right side and runs to the gall bladder. The continuation of the biliary tree distal to this point is the common bile duct. The common bile duct descends in the right anterior aspect of the free edge of the lesser omentum, and then passes posterior to the first part of the duodenum. It then lies in a groove in the posterior of the head of the pancreas. Usually it is joined by the main pancreatic duct, and together they open into the medial wall of the second part of the duodenum at the apex of the duodenal papilla (ampulla of Vater). The opening is guarded by a sphincter (Oddi). The gall bladder is a sac lying

190

on the right inferior aspect of the liver. It is divided into a fundus, body and neck, the last being continuous with the cystic duct. The cystic duct runs down the lesser omentum, eventually to fuse with the common hepatic duct and form the common bile duct. It is bound by peritoneum to the undersurface of the liver. Its function is to concentrate and store bile and to contract and release bile into the duodenum to promote digestion of a fatty meal.
[A:1310; B:399; G:281]

455 All the venous blood from the intestine and intestinal derivatives is gathered together in the hepatic portal vein for passage through the liver. In general, the foregut is drained by the splenic vein, midgut by the superior mesenteric vein and hindgut by the inferior mesenteric vein. The portal vein is usually formed posterior to the neck of the pancreas by the confluence of the superior mesenteric and splenic veins. The inferior mesenteric vein usually drains into the splenic vein some 3 cm to the left of this point. The portal vein passes upwards and to the right, posterior to the first part of the duodenum, to enter the free edge of the lesser omentum, where it ascends to the liver.
[A:710; C:636; E:205]

456 There are certain areas in the body where the portal and systemic veins come into contact. Venous blood may then drain into either the portal vein or the caval system. Obviously these portosystemic anastomoses will be situated at the superior and inferior ends of the intestine where the gut meets body wall. There are other sites, however, where bowel is deficient of peritoneal covering and around the umbilicus.

Clinically, the most important anastomosis is at the lower part of the oesophagus where tributaries of the left gastric vein (portal system) communicate with oesophageal veins draining to the azygos system. There is a similar anastomosis at the anus where superior rectal veins (tributaries of the inferior mesenteric vein) anastomose with inferior rectal veins (tributaries of iliac veins). There are also anastomoses between the two systems behind the ascending and descending colon, pancreas and duodenum, and the bare area of the liver (i.e. organs

which have lost their mesenteries and are in contact with the posterior abdominal wall). The paraumbilical veins run in the falciform ligament. They form a portosystemic anastomosis by connecting the left branch of the portal vein with superficial veins of the anterior abdominal wall.
[A:712; B:418; D:92; E:205]

E Applied answers

457 A common approach to liver biopsy is through the right eighth or ninth intercostal space in the mid-axillary line. Having passed through skin and superficial structures (including the intercostal muscles), the needle pierces the costal parietal pleura, crosses the costodiaphragmatic recess, through the diaphragmatic pleura and into the diaphragm. The needle now moves on respiration and the liver is biopsied in a quick 'one second' jab, the patient holding his breath in expiration. As both pleurae are normally pierced, a pneumothorax is an obvious potential hazard.
[D:58; E:125]

458 When the biopsy needle is in the liver substance, the diaphragm must remain static; otherwise the liver will move and be lacerated by the needle.
[A:1257; D:58; E:125]

459 Riedel's lobe is a tongue-like extension of the right lobe of the liver and may even extend into the pelvis. It is thought to be a congenital abnormality, though tight lacing in women was once suggested as a causative factor! Its clinical significance is that although itself it is of no pathological significance, it may easily be mistaken for a tumour of the liver, omentum, pancreas or even a distended gall bladder.
[A:1306; J:212]

460 The portal venous system is most easily seen by performing a splenoportogram x-ray. This can be obtained by percutaneous splenic puncture, operative mesenteric venography or via a selective splenic arteriogram. Most commonly, a percutaneous approach combined with splenic

manometry is used in the investigation of portal hypertension. Following contrast injection, the vascular tree and especially the splenic, superior mesenteric and portal veins are demonstrated, followed by a 'hepatogram' showing the intrahepatic venous tree. This technique may be used to see collaterals in cirrhosis, with oesophageal varices or to check the patency of a previous portacaval shunt.
[H:230; J:212]

461 A gallstone ileus usually happens due to previous inflammation of the gall bladder, causing it to adhere to its anterior relation, the duodenum. Later, the inflamed gall bladder, containing stones, ruptures or ulcerates into the duodenum and deposits its stony contents into the duodenum. A large stone may thus find itself obstructing the small bowel.
[A:1310; D:104]

462 The pain of biliary disease may be localised to the right subcostal margin or quite commonly is felt as referred pain to the right shoulder or the inferior tip of the right scapula. The gall bladder receives branches from the anterior and posterior hepatic plexi. The afferent nerve supply is believed to pass via sympathetics through the splanchnic nerves and the right phrenic nerve. This phrenic connection is thought to explain the referred pain of the right shoulder in the region of the C4 dermatome.
[A:1311]

463 A known history of gallstones and a sudden onset of jaundice makes one think that the stones have been expelled from the gall bladder, passed along the cystic duct and into the common bile duct where they have caused an obstruction to the flow of bile. The normal width, as seen on x-ray, of the common bile duct is not greater than 12 mm, so a couple of medium-sized stones can easily obstruct it, especially at the sphincter of Oddi. Work on the detailed musculature of the sphincter has shown that there is sometimes both a pancreatic and a bile duct sphincter (Boyden) as well as the combined ampullary sphincter of Oddi.
[F:222; G:288]

F Information answers

464 The right kidney is situated at a slightly lower
level than the left and, owing to the asymmetry
of the abdominal contents, the anterior relations on the two sides are different. The difference in height of the two organs accounts for
minor differences in the posterior relations. The
latter will, for the sake of ease of description, be
ignored. The posterior relations of the kidneys
are the diaphragm, the costodiaphragmatic
recess of the pleura, the twelfth rib, psoas,
quadratus lumborum and transversus abdominis. The subcostal nerve (T12) and iliohypogastric and ilioinguinal nerves (L1) are also posterior relations. The anterior relations of the right
kidney (from top to bottom) are the right suprarenal gland, liver, right colic flexure and second
part of duodenum, and small intestine. The
anterior relations of the left kidney (from top to
bottom) are the left suprarenal gland, stomach
and spleen, tail of the pancreas, left colic flexure
and small intestine.
[A:1316; D:112; F:233]

465 The kidneys are closely invested by a true
fibrous capsule. Outside this capsule is a layer
of fat—the perinephric fat. This fat is in its turn
enclosed by the renal fascia which also surrounds the suprarenal gland. The kidney therefore is surrounded by three fascial layers:
capsule proper, perinephric fat and renal fascia.
[A:1320; C:644; E:220]

466 In development, the kidney is initially situated
in the pelvis, the blood supply being derived
from the nearest available artery—usually the
common iliac artery. The kidneys ascend up the
posterior abdominal wall, their blood supply
migrating with them so that finally the renal
arteries arise from the aorta at the level of L1.
Sometimes the pelvic position may persist or
the kidney may be arrested in its ascent. The
renal artery in those instances would be derived
either from the common iliac arteries or from
the aorta near to its bifurcation.
[A:185; D:117; G:2113]

467 Both renal veins drain into the inferior vena
cava at the level of the transpyloric plane (L1).

However, asymmetry occurs as a result of drainage of the gonadal veins. On the right, this vein usually drains directly into the inferior vena cava, below the level of the renal vein. On the left, the gonadal vein usually drains into the left renal vein.
[A:659, 710; D:129; G:299]

468 From the minor calices urine flows into one of two or three major calices. These coalesce to form the pelvis of the kidney. Urine flows into the major calices and then through a constriction—the pelviureteric junction—into the ureter, down which it flows. The ureter is 25 cm long and runs downwards vertically behind the peritoneum on psoas, in line with the tips of the lumbar transverse processes. The ureter enters the pelvis by crossing the bifurcation of the common iliac artery, anterior to the sacroiliac joint where a narrowing may be present as it passes over the pelvic brim. It then runs downwards and backwards to the region of the ischial spine, where it turns forwards and medially to enter the bladder. It traverses the bladder wall in an oblique manner, this intramural part being the narrowest point of the ureter. Urine is propelled down the ureter into the bladder by peristalsis. Calculi may become lodged at any of the three narrow sites mentioned above. It should be said that the relations of the abdominal ureter are different on the two sides but the same in the two sexes, whereas the relations of the pelvic ureter are the same on the two sides but different in the two sexes.
[A:1319; D:116; G:299, 2110]

469 The arterial supply to the ureters is derived from different vessels as the ureter descends. Being adherent to the peritoneum, vessels eventually reach the ureter via the peritoneum. Superiorly, in the abdomen, these vessels are derived from the renal artery, lower down from the gonadal artery. In the pelvis, blood is obtained from the superior vesical artery. Venous blood drains to corresponding veins.
[A:1329; C:651]

470 The hilum of the kidney transmits—from anterior to posterior—the renal vein, the renal artery and the ureter.
[A:1317; B:410; H:239]

471 The right suprarenal gland is pyramidal and is situated on the upper pole of the right kidney. Anterior to it is the right lobe of the liver, and its medial extremity lies behind the inferior vena cava. Posterior to it is the diaphragm. The left suprarenal gland is crescentic and is situated on the superomedial aspect of the left kidney, extending almost as far inferiorly as the hilum. Anterior to it are the pancreas and lesser sac and stomach. Posterior to it is the diaphragm. [A:1378; C:643; G:299]

472 A trick question to which I hope you didn't fall! There is no connection whatsoever between the sympathetic nervous system and the adrenal cortex, except perhaps for some vasomotor fibres supplying the blood vessels. The cortex is the site of steroid production. The connection is with the adrenal medulla. Preganglionic sympathetic fibres from the splanchnic nerves run to the medulla where they synapse. The cells of the medulla are modified postganglionic cells. They release their catecholamines into the circulation. [A:1381; C:646; G:2114]

F Applied answers

473 Left-sided varicoceles are sometimes thought to be due to the fact that the loaded sigmoid colon lies anterior to the left testicular vein. Partial obstruction of this vessel will lead to varicosities of the pampiniform plexus, a varicocele. Another anatomical explanation is that the left testicular vein drains into the left renal vein at an angle of about 90°, and any slight alteration in the angle of confluence may cause obstruction. However, haematuria with a palpable abdominal mass must make one suspicious of a renal mass. Classically, adenocarcinoma of the kidney spreads directly along the renal vein, and thus the tumour will obstruct testicular venous flow and cause haematuria and an enlarged left kidney. [A:710; D:129; E:167]

474 Different methods are used to locate the exact position for renal biopsy, but most of them involve the use of x-rays and markers on the

patient's skin of the back. The needle pierces in succession the skin, superficial fascia and the posterior layer of the lumbar fascia, and usually runs through the lateral edge of the quadratus lumborum muscle. It then passes through the anterior lumbar fascia and paranephric fat and is cautiously advanced until it lies in the renal fascia. Similar in method to a liver biopsy, the needle is advanced through the renal fascia and perinephric fat only when the patient holds his breath in inspiration. The operator must not hold the needle while the patient breathes; it must be allowed to swing freely, otherwise lacerations may occur.
[A:1316; D:59]

475   The surface markings of the kidney are most easily drawn on the back and overlie the erector spinae medially and quadratus lumborum laterally. Bearing in mind that they move about 2 cm inferiorly during inspiration, the upper pole lies opposite the T11 or 12 spine, the lower pole opposite the spine of L3. The hila of the kidneys are opposite the first lumbar vertebra. Due to the liver mass, the right kidney is normally slightly lower than the left, and the right lower pole may just be palpated in a thin subject on full inspiration.
[B:407; C:643; D:59]

476   The posterior relations of both kidneys include the diaphragm and the costodiaphragmatic recess of the pleural cavity. A biopsy involving any part but the lower poles might well pierce both layers of the pleura and cross the recess and thus expose the patient to a risk of pneumothorax.
[A:1316; D:59]

477   A horseshoe kidney is a developmental abnormality caused by the fusion of the two metanephric masses and is found more commonly in men than in women. The normal kidney migrates cranially but the horseshoe kidney cannot because vessels such as the inferior mesenteric artery prevent such ascent. Often the single kidney receives its blood supply from the iliac artery, and, due to malrotation of the pelves, ureteric obstruction is a frequent problem. Variants of this abnormality include a

pelvic cake or central 'lump' kidney and the S-shaped kidney, both of which have anteriorly placed pelves and anomalous vasculature.
[A:183; G:2113]

478 Plain radiography may occasionally reveal the outline of the calyces and renal pelvis, particularly if a staghorn calculus is present. However, the more conventional techniques of intravenous pyelography (urography) and retrograde pyelography give a much clearer picture. During a urogram it is normal to take a plain abdominal film prior to intravenous contrast injection. Following the injection, ureteric compression is often used to show better renal filling and films taken at intervals (e.g. 10, 15, 20, 30 minutes) demonstrate the passage of contrast from kidney to bladder.
[J:72, 260]

479 As seen on a plain x-ray, the right ureter lies between the hilum of the kidney and the sacroiliac joint. It descends posterior to the parietal peritoneum on the psoas major muscle which separates it from the lower lumbar vertebral transverse processes. It is a vertical line down these processes which marks out the pathway of the ureter.
[D:117; E:243; J:72]

480 There are three relatively narrow parts of the ureter at which calculi tend to lodge. These are the pelviureteric junction (PUJ), where the pelvis forms the descending abdominal ureter; the pelvic brim just anterior to the sacroiliac joint; and the ureteric orifice which traverses the bladder wall obliquely. This last is the narrowest site of all.
[B:464; C:651; D:116]

G Information answers

481 The lumbar plexus is situated within the psoas muscle. The definitive nerves leave psoas laterally, medially or anteriorly. Those which leave psoas on its lateral border—from superior to inferior—are the iliohypogastric (L1), ilio-

inguinal (L1), the lateral cutaneous nerve of the thigh (L2, 3) and the femoral nerve (L2, 3, 4). [A:1050; B:425; G:2119]

482 The aorta enters the abdomen by running behind the diaphragm at T12. It descends on the bodies of the lumbar vertebrae and terminates at L4 by bifurcating into the common iliac vessels. Its paired branches can be divided into those supplying viscera and those supplying the body wall. The visceral branches are three—the renal artery, gonadal artery and suprarenal artery. The body wall vessels are five—the inferior phrenic and four lumbar arteries. For the sake of completeness, it should be remembered that the aorta has three midline unpaired gut branches: the coeliac, superior mesenteric and inferior mesenteric arteries. It also has an unpaired body wall vessel which arises at the aortic bifurcation—the median sacral artery.
[A:659; B:414; F:240; G:23]

483 The inferior vena cava commences in front of the body of L5, behind the right common iliac artery, by the union of the two common iliac veins. It ascends on the right side of the aorta, passes anterior to the right renal artery and runs in a groove on the posterior surface of the liver. It pierces the central tendon of the diaphragm to reach the thorax, and after a short intrathoracic course drains into the right atrium. It receives at its commencement the median sacral vein. As it ascends, it receives body wall tributaries symmetrically from each side—the inferior phrenic and four lumbar veins. It receives symmetrically the two renal veins at the level of L1 and three hepatic veins as it passes through the liver substance.

Because it is situated to the right of the midline, some of its tributaries are asymmetrical. Thus it receives the right gonadal vein and the right suprarenal vein directly. On the left, these vessels drain into the left renal vein.
[A:708; C:664; E:226; G:299]

484 The hypogastric plexus is a plexus of autonomic nerves. It is situated retroperitoneally in the lower abdomen and pelvis, anterior to the lower part and bifurcation of the abdominal

199

aorta, and between the common iliac arteries—a right and left branch supplying each side. The part in relation to the aorta is sometimes called the superior hypogastric plexus, the part between the common iliac vessels the inferior hypogastric plexus.

The sympathetic input to the plexus is from downward prolongations of the aortic plexus and branches from adjacent ganglia of the sympathetic chain. The parasympathetic input is from the pelvic splanchnic nerves (S2, 3, 4). The plexus supplies pelvic viscera with autonomic nerves by sending branches which run with blood vessels.

[A:1079; B:456; E:230; G:2114]

485 The lymph nodes of the posterior abdominal wall are distributed around the aorta. Preaortic nodes are situated anterior to the aorta, para-aortic nodes to the right and left sides. The preaortic nodes receive the lymph from the intestine. The lymph from the gut follows the intestinal arteries to the aorta. The preaortic lymph nodes are therefore situated around the origins of the coeliac, superior mesenteric and inferior mesenteric arteries. Efferent lymph from these nodes drains upwards as the intestinal trunk. The para-aortic nodes receive lymph from the kidneys, gonads and suprarenals. They also receive lymph from the deep layers of the abdominal walls and from their respective common iliac nodes. The lymph drains superiorly to the right and left lumbar trunks. The intestinal trunk and the lumbar trunks drain to the cisterna chyli, just below the aortic opening in the diaphragm.

[A:740; E:228]

486 The relationship of structures at the pelvic brim may be easily determined if one knows that structures concerning the body wall are posterior to structures concerning the genitourinary system and that, within the genitourinary system, genital structures are anterior to urinary structures. Thus at the pelvic brim the common iliac artery is the most posterior structure. It bifurcates as it crosses the pelvic brim into external and internal iliac arteries. The ureter crosses anterior to this bifurcation to reach the pelvis. The testicular vessels, having in their

turn crossed the ureter anteriorly in the abdomen to gain its lateral side, cross the external iliac artery at the brim lateral to the ureter.
[A:666; F:240; G:351]

487 In order to answer questions concerning the relationships of structures in the posterior abdominal wall, it is necessary to realise that various organ systems bear a constant relationship to each other. Any structure concerning the gastrointestinal tract is anterior to any structure concerning the genitourinary tract, which in turn is anterior to any structure concerning the body wall. Furthermore, structures concerning the genital tract are anterior to structures concerning the urinary tract.

Thus psoas will be the most posterior structure on our list. The ureter runs down subperitoneally on psoas. During its descent on psoas, it will be crossed anteriorly by the testicular vessels running from medial to lateral. The left ureter and testicular vessels will have no relationship with the right colic artery. The right testicular vessels (and the ureter, which is posterior to them) will be crossed by the right colic artery, which is therefore the most anterior of all these structures.
[A:666; F:240; G:299]

488 The origin of the diaphragm may be divided into three parts: a sternal part, a costal part and a vertebral part. These fibres arise circumferentially about the margin of the body wall and are inserted into a three-leaf-clover-shaped central tendon.

The sternal part consists of small slips which arise from the internal aspect of the xiphisternum. The costal part comprises slips which arise from the internal aspects of the lower six ribs, interdigitating with transversus abdominis.

The vertebral part consists of two crura—left and right. The right crus is the larger and arises from the right side of the bodies of L1–3. The left crus arises from the left side of the bodies of L1 and 2. The right crus is supposed to be the larger because the liver gives more resistance to diaphragmatic descent on that side. Posterolaterlly, the medial and lateral arcuate ligaments which are condensations over posas and

quadratus lumborum muscles also act as diaphragmatic origins.
[A:516; D:13; G:2120]

489 The median, medial and lateral arcuate ligaments are situated where the diaphragm is in contact with the posterior body wall. The median arcuate ligament is a fibrous connection between the medial borders of the two crura. The aorta runs behind this ligament. The medial arcuate ligament is situated lateral to the median arcuate ligament. It is the thickened upper margin of the fascia covering the anterior aspect of psoas. It extends from the upper part of the body of L2 to the transverse process of L1. Similarly, the lateral arcuate ligament is a thickening in the fascia covering the anterior aspect of quadratus lumborum. It is situated lateral to the medial arcuate ligament and extends from the tip of the transverse process of L1 to the lower aspect of the twelfth rib.
[A:516; D:13; E:587]

490 The central tendon of the diaphragm is formed from the septum transversum (which also forms the connective tissue of the liver) situated under the heart. The body wall sends a process inwards, one from each side, to meet the septum transversum. This is the pleuroperitoneal membrane. It eventually meets the septum transversum, with which it fuses. It then turns upwards as the pleuropericardial membrane, to separate the heart from the lung. This portion eventually becomes the fibrous pericardium. The fusion of the septum transversum and the pleuroperitoneal membranes leaves a gap posteriorly. This is filled by mesentery cells from the oesophagus. The muscle of the diaphragm is derived from cervical somites which migrate to invade the connective tissue skeleton. This explains why the phrenic nerve (C3, 4, 5) supplies the diaphragm. The pleuroperitoneal membrane brings its own nerve supply with it as it migrates. Thus a rim of the diaphragm is supplied by sensory fibres from the lower six intercostal nerves.
[A:182; C:655; G:2121]

491 There are three principal openings in the diaphragm: the caval opening, the oesophageal opening and the aortic opening.

The caval opening is at the level of T8. It is in the central tendon of the diaphragm, which acts to keep the vena cava open during all phases of the respiratory cycle. It transmits the inferior vena cava and terminal branches of the right phrenic nerve.

The oesophageal opening is at the level of T10, being 2.5 cm to the left of the midline. The oesophagus, vagus nerves, branches of the left gastric vessels and lymphatics are transmitted through this orifice. Its boundaries are muscular, as it runs through the left crus. However, a sling of fibres from the right crus cross the midline and loop round it, thus reinforcing the opening.

The aortic opening is at the level of T12 and is situated between the crura, which are bridged by the median arcuate ligament. Thus in reality this opening is behind the diaphragm. The aortic opening transmits the aorta, thoracic duct and azygos vein.

In addition to the above openings, other structures pass directly through the diaphragm. Thus the splanchnic nerves (greater, lesser and least) pierce the crura. The sympathetic trunks pass behind the medial arcuate ligament on the psoas muscle. The subcostal nerve and vessels run behind the lateral arcuate ligament. The left phrenic nerve pierces the dome to the left of the midline, to supply the diaphragm from its abdominal surface. The superior epigastric vessels pass between the sternal and costal origins. Lastly the neurovascular bundles of T7–11 pass between the digitations of the diaphragm and the transversus abdominis to reach the abdominal wall.

[A:516; B:267; D:13; G:2120]

G Applied answers

492 The coeliac ganglia are numerous nodular masses joined by variable connections to form the star-shaped coeliac plexus (solar plexus). It is the largest autonomic plexus and lies around the origin of the coeliac arterial trunk and on the crus of the diaphragm. The superior mesenteric ganglion lies at the inferior margin of the plexus. The coeliac plexus receives sympathetic contributions from the three splanchnic nerves

of the thorax and via the first lumbar ganglia. Parasympathetic connections are mainly from the posterior vagal trunk and some smaller nerves from the anterior vagus. The vagus controls the bowel as far as the splenic flexure. This immensely rich nervous input means that a direct blow to the solar plexus causes rapid changes in gut blood flow, leaving the victim with a feeling of impending doom and very 'winded'.
[A:1077; C:671; G:2114]

493 Tuberculosis of the spine (Pott's disease) is often seen as a paravertebral abscess in the thoracolumbar region. The pus may then track laterally under the fascia of the psoas muscle (psoas sheath) and, in doing so, may later appear as a fluctuant swelling below the inguinal ligament in the groin. The psoas abscess is easily mistaken for a femoral hernia.
[D:160; E:171]

494 The cisterna chyli is best seen on a first day (24 h) abdominal lymphangiogram. It is found anterior to the bodies of L1 and 2, receiving vessels from the para-aortic glands and intestinal lymphatic trunks, and is thus the final collecting chamber of the lymphatics from the abdomen and lower limbs. It gives off the thoracic duct, which ascends posterior to the diaphragm and through the posterior mediastinum before opening into the left brachiocephalic vein.
[A:727; J:222]

495 The abdominal aorta lies in the midline and is often palpable in the epigastric region in the supine thin subject. Inferiorly, the aorta bifurcates to the left of the midline at the level of the iliac crests.
[B:414; F:238; H:236]

496 The testis drains lymph via the spermatic cord to the posterior abdominal wall from whence it developed. It normally drains to the para-aortic nodes lying between the level of the common iliac veins and renal veins.
[A:741; D:128]

497 The diaphragm is formed from four main parts: the septum transversum, which becomes the central tendon; the body wall tissues; the dorsal mesentery of the oesophagus; and the two pleuroperitoneal membranes, which close off the pleura from the peritoneal cavity. Congenital herniae are most commonly seen in the posterolateral portion of the pleuroperitoneal canal (foramen of Bochdalek). Less common are herniae in the retrosternal portion of the diaphragm (foramen of Morgagni). Defects in the left leaf of the diaphragm are much more common than in the right, and occasionally the whole central tendon fails to develop. Right leaf diaphragmatic abnormalities are often associated with other congenital defects. Oesophageal herniae are sometimes congenital but much more often are of an acquired nature. These latter are divided into the sliding and rolling types, and are classically found in middle-aged, overweight women due to a weakness of the phreno-oesophageal ligament. Rolling herniae are also termed 'paraoesophageal', as the cardia remains in its anatomical position, but the fundus of the stomach protrudes into the thoracic cavity alongside the oesophagus. Occasionally, the whole stomach herniates and produces an 'upside-down' stomach in the thoracic cavity.
[D:16, 182]

498 The diaphragm's motor supply is entirely from the two phrenic nerves (C3, 4 and 5) and its sensory supply is via both phrenic nerves and the lower intercostal nerves. The latter are only sensory to the peripheral portions of the diaphragm derived from the body wall. Central diaphragmatic pain is therefore referred to the dermatomes of the phrenic nerve and is felt over the upper shoulder region.
[B:269; C:657]

499 The inferior vena cava must pass through the central tendon because, during inspiration, the muscular portion of the diaphragm contracts and, should this compress the vena cava, then one would faint 15–18 times a minute due to reduced venous return. In fact, the central tendon holds open the vena cava and reduced

intrathoracic pressure causes the blood to be sucked towards the heart (*vis a tergo*).
[A:516; D:13]

PELVIS AND PERINEUM

A   Information answers

500   The pelvis is divided into two parts. The true pelvis lies below the pelvic brim, the false pelvis above. The pelvic brim is a line which can be followed round the inner circumference of an articulated pelvis and consists of the sacral promontory posteriorly, the iliopectineal lines laterally and the symphysis pubis anteriorly. The false pelvis forms part of the abdominal cavity. In the adult, the pelvic viscera are usually limited to the true pelvis.
[A:351; F:272; G:32]

501   The orientation of the pelvis in the anatomical position is with the pubic tubercles and anterior superior iliac spines in the same vertical plane. For convenience, a wall may make the ideal plane of reference.
[A:354; B:439; C:366; G:39]

502   The pelvic inlet is the line which demarcates the true pelvis from the false pelvis, and consists of the sacral promontory posteriorly, the iliopectineal lines laterally and the symphysis pubis anteriorly. It is an indistensible bony ring through which the fetal head must pass during labour. The pelvic outlet is bounded posteriorly by the coccyx, laterally by the ischial tuberosities and sacrotuberous ligaments, and anteriorly by the pubic arch. It is an incomplete osseoligamentous ring which is distensible and therefore its conjugates are not absolute, as it may be stretched during labour.
[A:351; B:441; E:269]

503   The symphysis pubis is a secondary cartilaginous joint. The articular surfaces of the bones are covered in hyaline cartilage and are held together by a disc of fibrocartilage between them. A small amount of movement is possible at this joint. The sacroiliac joints are synovial joints, involving the auricular surfaces of the ilium and

the ala of the sacrum. Like all synovial joints, these articular surfaces are covered in cartilage and the joint is reinforced by anterior and posterior sacroiliac ligaments and the accessory sacrotuberous and sacrospinous ligaments. The posterior ligaments are particularly strong; together with the interlocking of the irregular articular joint surfaces, they prevent all but the smallest movement at these joints.
[A:442, 444; B:444; E:282; F:275]

504 The inguinal ligament is the rolled-up free lower border of the external oblique aponeurosis and extends from the anterior superior iliac spine to the pubic tubercle. In the anatomical position, the superior pubic ramus lies behind and a little above the line of this ligament. The lacunar ligament extends from the pubic end of the inguinal ligament backwards and upwards to the superior pubic ramus. Laterally, it has a free sharp crescentic margin which forms the medial limit of the femoral ring. It is on this sharp edge that femoral herniae frequently become strangulated.
[A:520; C:573; G:210]

505 The female pelvis is modified to allow passage of the fetal head through the pelvic inlet, canal and outlet during labour. In order to do this the diameters of the inlet and outlet are increased. In the male, the greater sciatic notch subtends less than a right angle. In the female the coccyx is carried backwards by increasing this angle to 90°, thereby increasing the anteroposterior diameter of the pelvic outlet. Thus it can be said that the greater sciatic notch is L-shaped in women and J-shaped in men (L for Lucy, J for Johnny).
[A:355; B:441; D:137; F:298]

506 The differences in the bony pelvis between the two sexes arise because of two factors. First, the male is the stronger. His pelvis is more strongly built, with more pronounced muscular markings. Second, the female pelvis is wider as a modification for the passage of the fetus in labour.

In the female, the pelvic inlet is oval to allow passage of the fetal head. In the male, it is heart-shaped owing to the forward projection

of the sacral promontory. The pelvic canal in the female is short with almost parallel sides and no projections, to allow an easy birth. In the male it is long with tapering sides, and the ischial spines project into it. Thus in the female the subpubic angle is greater than 90°. In the male it is less than 90° and in the female the sciatic notch is L-shaped whereas in the male it is J-shaped. Furthermore, the inferior pubic rami are strong and everted in the male for the attachment of the crura penis; this marking is absent in the female.
[A:355; D:137; E:282]

A Applied answers

507 First of all, the ischial tuberosities are palpated, the woman usually lying in the lithotomy position, and an intradermal weal of local anaesthetic is produced half-way between the tuberosity and the rectum. With middle and index fingers in the vagina, the needle is guided just beyond and inferior to the palpable ischial spine, where local anaesthetic is injected. This blocks the main pudendal nerve as it passes dorsal to the spine prior to entering the pudendal canal (Alcock).
[B:501; D:157; H:257]

508 The true conjugate is the measurement from the sacral promontory to the upper and inner border of the pubic symphysis, whereas the diagonal conjugate is from the sacral promontory to the lower border of the symphysis.
[B:441; D:137]

509 The sacral hiatus is the bony landmark used for caudal epidural injections. Mainly used for back pain or during labour, epidural anaesthesia is achieved by introducing the needle through the sacrococcygeal ligament, traversing the sacral hiatus, and injecting the local anaesthetic in the space occupied by sacral roots and filum terminale.
[B:521; H:81]

510 These 'dimples of Venus' are the posterior superior iliac spines, often seen in a well nourished woman as dimples but in thin indi-

viduals only as two bony prominences. They are a useful guide as to the approximate level of the end of the thecal sac as well as the S2 vertebra and the midpoint of the sacroiliac joint. [B:546; H:267]

511 The subpubic angle is under the arch formed by the two ischiopubic rami and the pubic symphysis. In the male, this tends to be a sharp angle of about 60°. In the normal female gynaecoid type of pelvis, the angle is a more gentle arch of about 120–130°. Therefore, a woman with an acute subpubic angle has a more android pelvis and may indeed have problems during childbirth due to a reduced available outlet space. [B:442; J:74]

512 The distance between the ischial spines is the diameter of the pelvic cavity. The normal measurement for interischial diameter is about 11 cm, so a patient presenting with an 8 cm diameter is a strong candidate for obstruction in the mid-cavity during labour. Depending on the size of her baby, this woman might require a Caesarian section. [B:441; C:478; D:137]

513 Normal measurements of the brim or pelvic inlet are 11.5 cm for the anteroposterior diameter, 12.5 cm for the transverse diameter and 12 cm for the diagonal diameter. The anteroposterior measurement is the true conjugate diameter, the transverse is the widest part of the brim and the diagonal or oblique measurement is from sacroiliac joint to iliopectineal eminence. [B:441; D:137]

B Information answers

514 The superficial fascia of the anterior abdominal wall is divided into a superficial fatty layer (Camper's fascia) and a deeper membranous layer (Scarpa's fascia). Colles' fascia is the continuation of Scarpa's fascia in the perineum. It is attached anteriorly to the pubic arch and posteriorly to the free border of the perineal membrane. It sends prolongations into the penis and scrotum in the superficial fascia of these struc-

tures. Between Colles' fascia and the perineal membrane is the superficial perineal pouch.
[A:519, 530; E:338; F:258]

515 The pudendal nerve is a branch of the sacral plexus. In company with the internal pudendal vessels, it leaves the pelvis through the greater sciatic foramen and turns immediately over the ischial spine into the lesser sciatic foramen to enter the pudendal canal (Alcock). The first branch, the inferior rectal nerve, is given off almost immediately. This nerve runs medially and breaks up to supply the external anal sphincter, perianal skin and part of levator ani. As the remainder of the pudendal nerve approaches the urogenital triangle, it divides into two—the dorsal nerve of the penis (or clitoris) and the perineal nerve. The former traverses the deep pouch and supplies the penis (or clitoris). The latter runs in the superficial pouch and supplies the muscles of the urogenital triangle and the skin of the scrotum (or labia).
[A:670, 1060; F:264]

516 The male urethra is divided into three parts: prostatic, membranous and penile (spongy). As its name suggests, the prostatic part traverses the prostate gland. This part of the urethra lies in the pelvis. The membranous part passes through the urogenital (deep pouch) diaphragm; that is, from superior to inferior, the superior fascia of the urogenital diaphragm, the sphincter urethrae muscle and the inferior fascia of the urogenital diaphragm (perineal membrane). The penile part runs through the corpus spongiosus of the penis. The membranous and penile parts lie in the perineum superficial to the levator ani muscle.
[A:1334; D:121; F:285]

517 The deep perineal pouch (space) is a triangular-shaped space bounded superiorly by the superior fascia of the urogenital diaphragm and inferiorly by the inferior fascia of the urogenital diaphragm (perineal membrane). Anterolaterally these two fascial sheets are attached to the pubic arch and ischiopubic rami, which thus form the space's boundaries in this direction. Posteriorly, the space is bounded as the fasciae fuse along the free border of the urogenital

diaphragm. In both sexes the pouch contains the membranous urethra and, surrounding it, the sphincter urethrae muscle, plus the deep transverse perineal muscles, the dorsal nerve of the penis (clitoris) and the blood vessels to the penis (clitoris). In the male it also contains the bulbourethral glands (Cowper). In the female the vagina passes through the deep pouch, piercing the sphincter muscles as it does so.
[A:531; C:729; E:339]

518 The superficial perineal pouch lies between Colles' fascia inferiorly and the inferior fascia of the urogenital triangle (perineal membrane) superiorly. Posteriorly these two structures fuse. Laterally its boundary is where these two fascial sheets attach to the ischiopubic rami but anteriorly it is in free communication with the subScarpal area of the anterior abdominal wall. The pouch contains the root of the penis (clitoris) and the associated muscles. These are the ischiocavernosus, bulbospongiosus and superficial transverse perineal muscles, which help maintain erection of the penis (clitoris).
[A:530, 1346, 1364; B:495]

519 The urogenital triangle is formed by the symphysis pubis anteriorly and the diverging ischiopubic rami laterally. Its posterior border is an imaginary line passing through the two ischial tuberosities.
[A:529; B:496]

520 In the anatomical position the penis is erect, so the dorsum is that part which faces upwards and backwards. In the flaccid state this part faces anteriorly. This can cause confusion to the uninitiated!
[A:1347; E:341; F:260]

521 The perineal body is a fibromuscular common tendon situated in the midline 1 cm anterior to the anal canal and behind the vagina (in the female) or bulb of penis (in the male). Eight muscles converge and are attached to this point: the two superficial transverse perinei, bulbospongiosus, the two deep transverse perinei, the anterior fibres of the two levator ani muscles and fibres from the superficial external anal sphincter. In the female it is frequently dam-

211

aged during delivery; the resulting weakness of the pelvic floor may cause prolapse of the pelvic organs.
[A:530; C:496; E:339]

522 The bulbourethral glands (Cowper) are found only in the male. They are situated in the deep perineal pouch, one on either side of the urethra. Their ducts, however, pierce the inferior fascia of the urogenital diaphragm (perineal membrane) to enter the superficial pouch and enter the urethra in the bulb of the penis. They are homologous in the female with the greater vestibular glands (Bartholin). They lie one on each side under the posterior parts of the labia majora and bulbs of the vestibule. Their ducts empty into the vestibule immediately distal to the hymen.
[A:1364, 1350; C:737]

523 The superficial inguinal lymph nodes drain the following structures on their respective side:
Lower limb
Gluteal region
Anterior abdominal wall below the umbilicus
External genitalia and perineum
Lower half of the anal canal
Vagina below the hymen
Body of the uterus via lymphatics which run in the broad ligament.
It should be stressed that lymph from the testis does not drain to this group of nodes. The lymphatics from this structure follow its blood vessels to the para-aortic nodes. In a case of enlargement of the superficial inguinal nodes, all the structures above must be inspected to ascertain the site of the primary lesion.
[A:734; B:205]

B   Applied answers

524 On a lateral view of a male urethrogram, the site of the perineal membrane is at the point where the bulbous urethra narrows abruptly on becoming the narrow membranous portion.

The narrowing caused by the sphincter urethrae is just proximal to the perineal membrane.
[I:1035; J:264]

525 An inflamed Bartholin's gland is seen as a red swollen labium majus, especially in the posterior part of the vestibule. The gland itself is the size of a pea and lies under cover of the posterior part of the bulb of the vestibule just lateral to the vaginal wall. The ducts open through this wall at the level of the hymen.
[E:344; G:334]

526 The widest part of the male urethra, when distended, is the prostatic portion, which is approximately 3 cm long and fusiform in shape. Surprisingly, the narrowest part is the external urethral meatus, with the membraneous urethra (at the site of the perineal membrane) running a close second.
[E:331; G:327; H:248]

527 Ejaculation is caused by afferent nervous impulses from the glans penis, causing sympathetic discharge to the smooth muscle fibres of epididymis, ductus deferens, seminal vesicles and prostate gland. Joined by secretions from the bulbourethral glands, the semen is ejected from the penis by rhythmic contractions of the ischiocavernosus and bulbospongiosus muscles. The sympathetic nerves are from the L1–2 outflow and pass to the pelvic organs via the pelvic plexi and especially the hypogastric plexus or presacral nerve, which lies on the promontory of the sacrum. It is the concavity of the sacrum and its close relationship with the posterior rectal wall which may cause ejaculatory problems following lower rectal surgery, especially after the operation of abdominoperineal excision of rectum.
[E:343; F:62; J:264]

528 A ruptured perineal body or central tendon may have few immediate consequences if not repaired properly. However, women in later life are prone to develop herniation of pelvic contents, leading to prolapse of the uterus, a rectocele or cystocele. This is due to the fact that

the perineal body is an important anchor point for many perineal muscles.
[B:492; E:340; G:339; H:257]

529 Urine extravasated into the superficial pouch or space is limited superficially by the extent of Colles' fascia of the perineum whilst its deep limit is the perineal membrane itself. The urine is limited to the anterior triangle of the perineum as Colles' fascia terminates at the posterior margin of the urogenital diaphragm to which it is firmly attached. The urine therefore first fills the penis but then, unable to spread posteriorly or laterally due to the attachments of Colles' fascia, it tracks into the scrotum and upwards over the pubis and under Scarpa's fascia of the lower abdomen. Along the inguinal ligaments Scarpa's fascia is fixed to the fascia lata of the thigh and so the extravasated urine continues its upward path in the superficial fascia of the abdomen.
[E:130, 338]

530 Hypospadias is an abnormal opening in the urethral floor, accompanied by an absent external meatus, found in about 0.2 per cent of male babies. The different degrees of hypospadias include the external meatus opening in the glans, along the ventral aspect of penis, or even in the perineum at the base of the penis. It is due to a failure of the urogenital folds, which are 'zipped' together from the perineum towards the glans. A failure in this mechanism is an important factor in understanding hypospadias. This condition may be associated with hypogonadism, a cleft scrotum and small penis, and thus makes sexing of the child quite difficult.
[A:193; C:739]

531 A cystoscope, being a fairly heavy instrument, tends to pass along the floor of the urethra and so avoids the lacuna magna in the roof of the navicular fossa. The tip of the cystoscope is normally at an angle to the shaft to aid the passage between the spongy and membranous urethra, at which point the penis is normally pulled downwards between the thighs. It is at this point, at the perineal membrane, that the urethra is held firmly in position and the in-

strument is most likely to wedge and, if forced, may create a false urethral passage.
[D:121; E:331; G:339; H:248]

532   Circumcision is simply removal of the foreskin in the male. Special care must be taken when cutting the frenulum which joins the ventral part of the glans penis to the foreskin, as this contains a small but fairly constant artery. It is interesting to note that circumcision in the male is excellent prophylaxis against cancer of the penis. Female circumcision involving the clitoris and labia is still practised worldwide, and is a cause of obstetric problems.
[G:328; H:246]

C   Information answers

533   Together with coccygeus, the levator ani muscle forms the floor of the pelvic cavity or pelvic diaphragm. Levator ani consists of two parts —iliococcygeus and pubococcygeus. The latter is further subdivided into levator prostatae (sphincter vaginae), puborectalis and pubococcygeus proper. The iliococcygeus is misnamed, as in man it has nothing to do with the ilium. It arises from the ischial spine and the posterior part of a line of thickened fascia over the obturator internus muscle (arcus tendineus). It is inserted into the coccyx and the anococcygeal raphe. The pubococcygeus is at a slightly higher level than the iliococcygeus. It arises from the posterior surface of the pubis and adjacent part of the arcus tendineus. Medially is the levator prostatae (sphincter vaginae), a U-shaped sling passing behind the prostate (or vagina) into the perineal body. More laterally, the puborectalis forms a sling round the anorectal junction, blending with the deep external anal sphincter. More laterally still, the pubococcygeus proper is inserted into the coccyx and anococcygeal raphe. The muscle is innervated by the perineal branch of S4 and the inferior rectal nerve.
[A:528; E:275]

534   The ischiorectal fossae are wedge-shaped spaces on either side of the anal canal. Their lateral wall is the obturator internus muscle and

the ischial tuberosity, the roof is the levator ani muscle and the floor is skin. Anteriorly, each fossa extends deep to the urogenital diaphragm, on either side of the urethra. Medially, the fossae are separated by the anal canal. They have nothing to do with the rectum, which is superior to the levator ani; the name 'ischiorectal fossa' is thus a misnomer. The ischiorectal fossa is full of loosely arranged fat to allow distension of the anal canal during defaecation. [A:530; E:277]

535 As its name suggests, the external anal sphincter is situated outside the internal anal sphincter. The internal sphincter is a thickening of the circular muscle of the intestinal wall and is composed of smooth muscle. Therefore, its nerve supply is from the autonomic system via the pelvic plexi. The external anal sphincter is composed of striped muscle and is under voluntary control. It is divided into three parts: subcutaneous, superficial and deep. The subcutaneous part is a muscular ring with no attachments. The superficial part consists of fibres which are attached to the coccyx posteriorly and the perineal body anteriorly, and thus helps to anchor the anal canal. The deep sphincter is a ring of muscle which is fused to the puborectalis part of the levator ani, forming the anorectal ring. This structure is vital for continence. Being a voluntary muscle, the external sphincter is supplied by the somatic nervous system, the inferior rectal branch of the pudendal nerve.
[A:1293; D:89; E:334]

536 The mid-point of the anal canal represents the junction between hindgut and body wall. The blood supply of the region reflects this fact. The artery of the hindgut is the inferior mesenteric artery. Its continuation, the superior rectal artery, divides into left and right branches as it reaches the rectum. The right branch divides again into anterior and posterior divisions. These branches supply the rectum and upper part of the anal canal in the position 3, 7 and 11 o'clock with the subject in the lithotomy position. The inferior rectal artery (body wall artery) is a branch of the pudendal artery, there being one on each side. They supply the lower

216

half of the anal canal. The middle rectal artery —again one on each side—is a branch of the internal iliac arteries. They supply only the muscle wall of the rectum. The veins correspond to the arteries, the superior rectal draining to the inferior mesenteric and eventually portal vein, and the inferior rectal to the iliac vein via the internal pudendal. The anal canal, therefore, is a site of portosystemic venous anastomosis.
[A:1293; B:488; D:87]

537 The human rectum, unlike that of other animals, is not straight. The upper and lower parts sit in the midline but the central portion is thrown out to the left. Three 'bends' in the rectum are thus produced; from above downwards, they turn left, right and left. Inside the rectum the 'inside' of each bend is marked by a shelf protruding from the rectal wall into the lumen and produced by all the layers of the wall. These three 'shelves' are the transverse folds or rectal valves (Houston). Their function is unclear, but in sigmoidoscopy they cause a nuisance by obstructing the instrument.
[A:174, 1290; E:292]

C Applied answers

538 The pectinate line is the demarcation in the anal canal between the embryonic proctodeum (ectoderm) and the embryonic cloaca (endoderm). The hymen is the partition between the vagina and the vestibule. The pectinate line divides the systemic blood supply inferiorly from the portal venous supply superiorly, and in a similar manner the autonomic nervous plexi supply above this line whilst the somatic inferior haemorrhoidal nerves supply below. As with the pectinate line, so does the lymphatic drainage of the vagina have a watershed; below the hymen and the pectinate line the skin of the vagina and anus drain to the superficial inguinal lymph nodes whilst the upper vagina and anus drain to iliac nodes. Both the hymen and the pectinate line are embryonic watersheds with important clinical significance.
[A:176; B:489; F:258; G:342; H:248]

539 The exact position of an anal carcinoma will determine the direction of lymphatic spread. Though there is clinically some overlap, a tumour situated below the pectinate line will drain to the groin (superficial inguinal nodes) whilst one above the line will spread to the internal iliac nodes. These latter will of course require pelvic surgery to be examined histologically.
[B:489; H:248]

540 An imperforate anus is a failure of the proctodeum and cloaca to meet. The pectinate line probably represents the former site of the anal membrane, which normally breaks down during the seventh week allowing the rectum to open into the amniotic sac. This membrane lies at the top of the anal pit, which is lined by ectoderm and formed by a dorsal extension of the urogenital fold. This explains why a shallow anal pit may deceive the physician as to the presence of a patent anus.
[A:176; B:489; C:710]

541 In the male examination, the prostate and, occasionally, healthy seminal vesicles as well as the bulb of the penis may be felt anteriorly. The normal prostate is felt as two lateral lobes separated by a median sulcus; the spongy urethra may also be felt, especially if there is a catheter in situ. In the female, the cervix uteri or a retroverted uterus is easily palpated and may even be mistaken for a rectal neoplasm! The perineal body and, very occasionally, the ovaries, lying in the pouch of Douglas, are also palpated. In both sexes, the ischiorectal fossae and ischial spines lie laterally, whilst posteriorly the sacrum and coccyx are within reach. On withdrawing the finger, the anorectal ring is felt as a thick band of muscle.
[B:490; D:88; E:353]

542 Haemorrhoids or piles are varicosities of the superior haemorrhoidal (rectal) veins. These veins are part of the portal venous system and it is within this region that there is a portosystemic venous anastomosis. Blockage of the portal venous outflow due to cirrhosis of the liver will therefore cause the portal veins to find alternative venous channels. Thus a site of portosystemic venous anastomoses may readily open

up and develop numerous enlarged tortuous veins seen as varices in the oesophagus or haemorrhoids in the rectum. Injection of irritant solutions into haemorrhoids must be performed above the pectinate line and hence into a region innervated by the autonomic nervous plexi, which is painless. Injection below the pectinate line is very painful due to its somatic innervation and you may lose your patient's custom!
[B:489; D:89; E:350]

543 The lithotomy position is literally that used for 'cutting for stone'. In fact, it is lying supine with the legs abducted and raised in stirrups for easy access to the perineum. It is used mainly for gynaecological and anal procedures. In this rather undignified position the boundaries of the anal triangle are the coccyx and two ischial tuberosities, with the base of this triangle across the perineum between the tuberosities, the apex being the coccyx.
[G:316; H:256]

544 The major content of the ischiorectal fossa is dense lobulated fat. This is a common site of both abscess and fistula formation due to the medial border of the fossa being the anal canal. It is therefore possible for fistulae to track into the fossa and form an abscess deep in the fat. External injury in the perianal skin may also lead to deep-seated abscess formation in the fossae. In performing surgery on fistulae and abscesses in this region, it is most important to leave the anorectal ring intact to avoid faecal incontinence.
[D:89; E:352; G:319; H:257]

D Information answers

545 The ejaculatory ducts pierce the prostate gland and terminate in the prostatic urethra. Their openings are found one on each side on the urethral crest, within the opening of the utricle.
[A:1344; E:301]

546 The nerve supply to the bladder is from the autonomic system. The sympathetic nerves are derived from the sacral plexi, the parasympathetic from the pelvic splanchnic nerves (nervi

erigentes, S2, 3 4). The parasympathetics are facilitatory to the detrusor muscle, the sympathetic inhibitory. Pain fibres from the bladder run mainly with the parasympathetics. The sphincter urethrae is striated muscle under voluntary control and is supplied by the pudendal nerve (S2, 3, 4).

[A:1080, 1333; C:712; E:322]

547 The internal iliac artery is important because it supplies the viscera and walls of the pelvis. It arises at the bifurcation of the common iliac artery in front of the sacroiliac joint. It descends to the greater sciatic foramen, where it divides into anterior and posterior divisions. The anterior division gives rise mainly to visceral branches. These are the umbilical artery (which, when obliterated, forms the medial umbilical ligament), the superior and inferior vesical arteries to the bladder, the uterine artery, the middle rectal artery to the muscle of the lower rectum and the obturator artery. The anterior division ends in the internal pudendal and inferior gluteal arteries. The posterior division gives rise to parietal branches. These are the iliolumbar, lateral sacral and superior gluteal arteries.

[A:668; B:451; C:715]

548 The normal prostate is described as having two capsules, and the pathological gland three. Both statements are incorrect. The prostate has only one true capsule, which is a thin fibrous envelope round the gland. The false capsule outside the true capsule is separated from it by the prostatic venous plexus. It consists of thickened pelvic fascia. Pathologically, an adenoma of the prostate will compress the remainder of the gland against the true capsule. This rim of squashed tissue inside the true capsule is the pathological capsule of the prostate.

[A:1349; D:123; E:301]

549 For the purposes of description, the rectum may be divided into thirds: upper, middle and lower. The relationship of the peritoneum is different in each third. In the upper third the rectum is covered by peritoneum anteriorly and on both sides, and only posteriorly is it absent. In the middle third the peritoneum covers only

the anterior aspect of the rectum, leaving both sides and the posterior aspect deficient. In the lower third the rectum has no relationship with the peritoneum, as the latter has been reflected onto the anterior pelvic organs.
[A:1291; F:283]

550 The trigone is a smooth triangular area situated on the internal aspect of the posterior wall (base) of the bladder. The three angles of the trigone are the two ureteric orifices superolaterally and the internal urethral orifice inferiorly. Between the two ureteric orifices is a ridge of muscle—the interureteric bar. The trigone, unlike the rest of the organ, does not distend as it fills. Pain receptors are numerous in this region.
[A:1332; G:348]

551 The prostatic urethra is not circular in cross-section but rather is kidney-shaped, consisting of a posterior midline ridge with a gutter on either side. The gutters constitute the prostatic sinus; the ridge is the verumontanum or urethral crest.
[A:1334; E:301; G:348]

D Applied answers

552 The female genital duct is called the paramesonephric (Müllerian) duct. During male development most of this duct regresses, leaving only the appendix testes and prostatic utricle in the male adult. Both of these may develop pathologically, the utricle producing a cystic swelling in the region of the verumontanum, whilst the appendix may undergo torsion and be misdiagnosed as acute epididymitis or even appendicitis due to the location of referred pain.
[A:187; B:468; F:297]

553 The prostatic venous plexus receives the deep dorsal vein of the penis and drains into the vesicular and hypogastric veins; eventually these drain into the internal iliac veins. The plexus is both valveless and thin-walled, and it has been shown that there are connections with the vertebral venous plexus (Batson). It is suggested that the frequent spread of prostatic

221

malignancy to the vertebral column is through this connection.
[I:578; J:144]

554   The urethra passes through the prostate gland itself, this portion being the widest 3 cm of the male urethra. Enlargement of the gland, and in particular its median lobe, causes retention of urine due to compression of the urethra, as well as an urge to frequent micturition due to pressure on the bladder neck.
[D:124; E:301; H:248]

555   A normal vasogram will reveal the ductus deferens (vas deferens) coming from the scrotum and crossing the pelvic cavity. It will often also show the ampulla of the vas lying just medial to the seminal vesicle and the two ejaculatory ducts opening into the prostatic portion of the urethra at the level of the verumontanum.
[C:689; I:1059; J:264]

556   Pain located at the tip of the penis is often referred pain from the trigone of the bladder. As this pain is associated with the end of micturition and haematuria, it would be reasonable to suggest that it is due to a bladder stone irritating the trigone as the bladder empties.
[F:280; G:348]

557   In the adult, the bladder is a pelvic organ, rising up into the abdominal cavity only when fully distended. Its superior surface is clothed in peritoneum which is reflected onto the anterior abdominal wall. As the bladder fills and becomes increasingly distended, the peritoneum is progressively stripped from the anterior abdominal wall, resulting in an area of bladder lying in direct contact with the abdominal wall without any peritoneum or peritoneal cavity intervening. This fact is utilised in making a suprapubic catheterisation in the linea alba just above the pubic symphysis, which avoids entering the peritoneal cavity.
[C:681; E:296; F:278; H:251]

558   The size, shape and position of the bladder vary with the volume of urine it contains, but in the normal adult one would expect to palpate or to percuss it only if it is well distended. In babies

and young children, however, it tends to be a relatively superficial organ situated largely in the abdominal cavity.
[E:296; F:278]

E Information answers

559 The ovary is pulled into its adult position in the pelvis by the gubernaculum ovarii. It originally comes from the upper lumbar region and, as it descends, it brings its blood, nerve and lymphatic supplies with it. Thus in the adult the ovarian arteries arise from the abdominal aorta immediately below the origin of the renal arteries (L1–2). The ovarian veins normally drain on the right into the inferior vena cava and on the left into the left renal vein (at the level L1–2). Furthermore, the ovarian nerves are derived from the renal and aortic plexi and accompany the blood vessels into the pelvis.
[A:666, 1353; F:295]

560 The round ligament of the uterus and the ligament of the ovary are the remains of the gubernaculum. In the male the gubernaculum pulls the testis from the lumbar region into the scrotum. In the female the descent of the ovary is arrested in the pelvis, but the gubernaculum may still be seen running from the pelvis, through the inguinal canal and into the labium majus (the homologue of the scrotum).
[A:189; C:693; E:144; H:247]

561 The uterus is normally described as anteverted and anteflexed. The long axis of the uterus is normally at an angle of some 90° to the long axis of the vagina, the uterine cervix entering the anterior vaginal wall. This is termed anteversion. Furthermore, the body and fundus of the uterus form an angle of some 160° with the cervix so that the uterus sits snugly on the bladder (anteflexion). In a small percentage of normal women, as well as pathologically, these relationships may be lost. Retroversion involves the uterus pointing towards the rectum and the vaginouterine angle exceeding 180°. Reversal of the angle between cervix and body to greater than 180° would be termed retroflexion.
[A:1357; D:150; E:307]

562 The uterine tube is some 10 cm long. It is found in the upper free border of the broad ligament and connects the cavity of the uterus with the peritoneal cavity via its lumen. It consists of four parts; from lateral to medial—infundibulum, ampulla, isthmus and interstitial part. The infundibulum is the funnel-shaped lateral extremity; it terminates in a number of finger-like processes (fimbriae), one or more of which clasp the ovary. The ampulla is the dilated portion of the tube adjacent to the infundibulum, where normal fertilisation occurs. The isthmus is the narrowest part of the tube and is found just lateral to the uterus. The interstitial part of the tube is found passing through the uterine wall and joins the isthmus to the cavity of the uterus.
[A:1354; B:477]

563 The drainage of lymph from the uterus is different in the various regions of the organ, viz. fundus, body and cervix. The fundus sends its lymph, together with that from the uterine (Fallopian) tube and ovary, along the ovarian vessels to the para-aortic nodes. The body drains laterally via the broad ligament to the lateral wall of the pelvis and nodes lying next to the external iliac vessels, the external iliac nodes. Part of the lymph from the body drains along lymphatics in the round ligament of the uterus to the superficial inguinal nodes. The cervix drains laterally via the broad ligament to the external iliac nodes, posterolaterally with the uterine vessels to nodes around the internal iliac vessels and posteriorly via lymphatics in the rectouterine fold round either side of the rectum to the sacral nodes.
[A:741; B:459; D:152]

564 The urachus is the allantoic diverticulum running from the cloaca into the umbilical cord. In the adult it is represented as a fibrous strand running from the apex of the bladder to the umbilicus—the median umbilical ligament. In the fetus the umbilical artery runs, one on each side, from the anterior division of the internal iliac artery to the umbilicus. In the adult they are obliterated and the resulting fibrous strand is the medial umbilical ligament.
[A:190, 1330; H:209]

565 The broad ligament passes from the lateral margins of the uterus to the lateral pelvic walls, thus acting as a septum and dividing the pelvis into two. Between its leaves is fibroareolar tissue, and in its upper free border the broad ligament contains the uterine tube. The ovary is attached to the posterior aspect of the ligament, and the 'services' to the ovary run between the lateral pelvic wall and the ovary in the lateral part of the broad ligament, forming the suspensory ligament of the ovary. Between the ovary and tube the ligament contains the epoöphoron and paroöphoron, the remains of the Wolffian (mesonephric) duct. The ovarian and uterine vessels form an anastomosing network in the ligament adjacent to the tube and uterus. The broad ligament also contains the remnants of the gubernaculum.
[A:1361; B:481; G:359]

566 The cervix uteri enters the anterior wall of the vagina and extends a short distance into it. Thus the upper part of the vaginal lumen surrounds the cervix like a gutter. This is the fornix. Although a continuous structure, the fornix is descriptively divided into anterior, posterior and right and left lateral fornices for purposes of orientation. The posterior fornix is deeper than the anterior owing to the fact that the cervix enters the anterior vaginal wall and is usually anteflexed.
[A:1362; E:307; F:295]

567 In the male, the peritoneum passes from the anterior abdominal wall onto the superior surface of the bladder. It runs down the posterior surface of the bladder for a short distance and is then reflected onto the middle third of the rectum, forming the rectovesical pouch as it does so. It then runs superiorly to form the parietal peritoneum of the posterior abdominal wall.

In the female the uterus is interposed between bladder and rectum. The peritoneum therefore runs from bladder to uterus, forming the uterovesical pouch, and thence from uterus to rectum, forming the rectouterine pouch (Douglas).
[A:1259; G:310; H:255]

568 The uterus is supported by the levator ani muscle and various condensations of pelvic fascia containing muscle termed ligaments. The levator ani forms the bulk of the pelvic diaphragm and supports the pelvic viscera above it. It supports the uterus indirectly by supporting the vagina via condensations of fascia to the region of the cervix and the perineal body. The cardinal, pubocervical and uterosacral ligaments are situated above levator ani and are attached to the cervix and upper vagina. The cardinal ligament runs to the lateral pelvic wall on each side. The pubocervical ligaments run from the pubic bone, and skirt either side of the bladder neck to reach the cervix uteri. The uterosacral ligaments form two bands on the posterolateral aspect of the pouch of Douglas as they pass lateral to the rectum and attach to the lower sacrum.
[A:1361; D:156; E:312]

E Applied answers

569 During a vaginal examination it is theoretically possible to palpate a ureteric stone through the lateral fornices. It is here that the ureters lie in the base of the broad ligament just lateral to the vaginal and uterine arteries which anastomose along the upper vaginal walls.
[E:305; G:363; H:255]

570 Usually preceded by a speculum examination, a bimanual pelvic examination can feel the external os of the cervix, the fornices and can be used to assess the size, position and shape of the uterus. A normal ovary may often be felt but the uterine tubes are palpable only if enlarged or thickened by disease. Examination of the posterior fornix may also reveal any abnormalities in the pouch of Douglas and often a normal ovary. The size of the bony pelvis may also be assessed, and a narrowed diagonal conjugate diagnosed if the examining fingers can reach the sacral promontory.
[B:485; D:157; E:355]

571 Free 'overspill' into the pouch of Douglas is an important sign, indicating patent uterine tubes as distinct from loculated spill due to pelvic

inflammatory disease. The hysterosalpingo-gram is a commonly used test in the investigation of infertility.
[B:478; I:1077; J:266]

572 If an embryo is destined to become female, the mesonephric tubules degenerate into the vestigial paroöphoron and epoöphoron of the broad ligament. The mesonephric duct (Wolffian) remnants are the epithelial cysts from the broad ligament to the vestibule and are called the canals of Gartner. These may cause cystic swellings requiring surgery.
[A:187; F:297]

573 The amateur abortionist often does not know the close relationship of the posterior fornix with the pouch of Douglas. In most women the posterior vaginal wall is longer than the anterior wall and in a direct line with the posterior fornix, especially in the anteverted uterus. Hence the aborting instrument slides along the posterior wall, through the thin wall of the posterior fornix and directly into the peritoneal cavity, with resultant peritonitis.
[E:303; H:254]

574 At the time of ovulation some women experience intermenstrual pain (mittelschmerz) due to the stretching of the ovarian wall. This is experienced as referred pain to the dermatome of the innervation of the ovary. The ovary is supplied from T10 fibres and so the pain is paraumbilical (cf. testis).
[G:358; H:255]

575 To explain an abdominal pregnancy one must realise that the ovum is expelled into the peritoneal cavity, only later to be diverted into the uterine tube by the fimbriae. If, as very rarely happens, the ovum is fertilised inside the peritoneal cavity by a sperm which has swum out of the peritoneal opening near the fimbria, then implantation can occur inside the peritoneal cavity. The other, more likely, occurrence is that during an abortion or rupture of a tubal ectopic pregnancy, the trophoblast reimplants itself in the broad ligament or pelvic peritoneal cavity. These abdominal pregnancies may

proceed to near term before they are discovered.
[G:367; H:255]

576 The uterus is supported or suspended by three groups of ligaments: the pubocervical anteriorly, the cardinal (Mackenrodt) laterally and the uterosacral posteriorly. These ligaments also help maintain the uterus in its correct position. Their stretching may lead not only to retroversion but, if they are not strong enough to counterbalance increases in intra-abdominal pressure, also to a gradual descent of the uterus. This can result in a complete prolapsed uterus (procidentia).
[B:480; C:701; H:255]

577 The lymphatic drainage of the ovary is to the para-aortic nodes on the posterior abdominal wall at the level of the renal vessels.
[B:459; J:226]

LOWER LIMB

A Information answers

578 The greater and lesser sciatic notches are converted into foramina by the sacrotuberous and sacrospinous ligaments. The sacrotuberous ligament is very strong. It is attached to the posterior inferior iliac spine and the lateral part of the sacrum and coccyx. It runs to the ischial tuberosity. It is supposed to be the phylogenetically degenerated tendon of the long head of biceps femoris. The sacrospinous ligament lies on the pelvic aspect of the sacrotuberous ligament and is triangular in shape. Its base is attached to the lateral aspect of the sacrum and coccyx, and its apex to the ischial spine. Phylogenetically it is the degenerated posterior aspect of coccygeus. These ligaments are important for the stability of the pelvis for they prevent the backward rotation of the sacrum when the upright posture is assumed.
[A:443; C:374; F:322; G:436]

579 The structures which exit from the pelvis and enter the gluteal region through the greater sciatic foramen below the piriformis muscle are

the sciatic nerve, the nerve to quadratus femoris, the inferior gluteal nerve and vessels, the posterior cutaneous nerve of the thigh, the nerve to obturator internus and the internal pudendal nerve and vessels. The sciatic nerve curves laterally and downwards to pass midway between the ischial tuberosity and greater trochanter into the thigh. The sciatic nerve hides the nerve to quadratus femoris, a branch of the sacral plexus which also supplies the inferior gemellus. The inferior gluteal nerve (L5, S1, 2) arises from the dorsal divisions of the sacral plexus and supplies gluteus maximus, accompanied by the inferior gluteal vessels. The posterior cutaneous nerve of the thigh supplies skin in the gluteal region and back of the thigh and leg. The nerve to obturator internus crosses the ischial spine and enters the ischiorectal fossa via the lesser sciatic foramen. It supplies obturator internus and the superior gemellus. The pudendal nerve and internal pudendal vessels also cross the ischial spine, medial to the nerve to obturator internus, to enter the ischiorectal fossa for distribution.
[A:444, 672, 1057; C:383; E:502; F:323; G:433]

580 Three structures leave the pelvis via the greater sciatic foramen, cross the ischial spine and enter the ischiorectal fossa by entering the lesser sciatic foramen. They are the pudendal nerve, the internal pudendal vessels and the nerve to obturator internus from medial to lateral.
[A:1060; C:383; E:502; F:323; G:433]

581 The sciatic nerve is derived from roots L4–S3 of the sacral plexus. It leaves the pelvis via the greater sciatic foramen below the piriformis muscle, to lie in the gluteal region. It curves downwards and laterally into the thigh, passing half-way between the ischial tuberosity and greater trochanter, lying successively on the superior gemellus, obturator internus, inferior gemellus and quadratus femoris. In the thigh it lies on adductor magnus, passing deep to the long head of biceps femoris. In the lower third of the thigh it divides into the tibial nerve, which passes medially, and the common peroneal nerve, which passes laterally. The tibial nerve is derived from ventral divisions of the

229

sciatic plexus, the common peroneal from dorsal divisions.
[A:1056; C:414; E:279; G:433]

582 The ligaments of the hip joint are the three capsular ligaments joining the innominate bone with the femur (iliofemoral ligament, ischiofemoral ligament and pubofemoral ligament) and two others—the transverse acetabular ligament and the ligamentum teres.

The strong iliofemoral ligament (Bigelow) is the shape of an inverted Y. Its base is attached to the anterior inferior iliac spine and its two limbs to the intertrochanteric line on the anterior of the femur. The ischiofemoral ligament forms a spiral between the ischium and the greater trochanter. The pubofemoral ligament is triangular. Its long base is attached to the superior pubic ramus, the apex to the inferior part of the intertrochanteric line.

The transverse acetabular ligament is formed by the labrum acetabulare as it spans the acetabular notch, converting it into a tunnel. The ligamentum teres is covered in synovial membrane. It runs between the pit of the head of the femur and the acetabular notch. It transports a small blood vessel to the head of the femur.

Extension of the hip to 15° results in tightening of the iliofemoral ligament, which therefore limits extension to this degree.
[A:446; C:416; F:364; G:442]

583 The principal abductors of the hip are gluteus medius and gluteus minimus. Tensor fascia lata and sartorius also abduct the hip, among other actions. If the hip bone is fixed, the gluteus medius and minimus will abduct the whole limb. If, however, the femur is fixed, the pelvis will be tilted towards the side of the contracting muscles, thereby reversing the role of origin and insertion. This movement is vital in walking. If the right leg is taken off the ground, the pelvis tends to fall to the unsupported right side. The left abductors contract, however, tilting the pelvis to the left and counteracting this drop. In fact, they overcompensate so that the pelvis is tipped a little to the left. This allows the right foot to clear the ground as the limb is swung forwards in taking a pace.
[A:449, 567; C:419; D:245; F:367]

584 The small lateral rotator muscles of the hip are: piriformis, obturator internus and its two gemelli, quadratus femoris and obturator externus.

Piriformis (a pear-shaped muscle) arises from the anterior surface of the second, third and fourth sacral vertebrae. It passes through the greater sciatic notch to its insertion on the greater trochanter. It forms a convenient reference point for other structures in the gluteal region. Obturator internus arises from the pelvic aspect of the obturator membrane and the surrounding bone. Its tendon passes through the lesser sciatic foramen, a bursa intervening as it winds round the ischium, and onto the greater trochanter. The gemelli, superior and inferior, run above and below the obturator internus tendon to the greater trochanter; the superior arises from the spine of the ischium, the inferior from the ischial tuberosity. The square quadratus femoris arises from the ischial tuberosity and inserts on the quadrate tubercle on the intertrochanteric crest of the femur. With the obturator internus and gemelli above it, it forms a 'bed' for the sciatic nerve. Obturator externus arises from the outside of the obturator membrane and the surrounding ischium and pubis. Its tendon is inserted into a pit on the medial aspect of the greater trochanter.
[A:568; C:383; F:325; G:434]

A Applied answers

585 The patient lies prone, or on his side, with the buttock muscles relaxed. The safe area for injection, if the buttock is to be used at all, is situated in the upper outer quadrant of the true anatomical buttock, and not just of the 'cosmetic' buttock! This is best located by marking a line from the greater trochanter of the femur to the dimple which marks the posterior superior iliac spine. Above this line is a safe area, and the lateral part of this region is often used for intramuscular injections. Nowadays, due to the dangers of hitting the sciatic or even the gluteal nerves, the tensor fasciae latae or vastus lateralis muscles are often the sites of choice, particularly in an unco-operative patient.
[D:231; H:293]

586 If the L4/5 disc has prolapsed, the nerve most likely to be affected is the L5 nerve root. Similarly, L5/S1 disc protrusion is most likely to cause problems with the S1 nerve root. Remember that in this region the spinal nerves exit from the intervertebral foramina below their numbered vertebral body, but usually above the level of the intervertebral disc, so that the more common lateral protrusions affect the spinal nerve below, whereas larger midline posterior disc protrusions may affect three or more of the lower roots. The pain will be worst in the same dermatomes, and these may show loss of sensation.

The L5 dermatome involves the lateral thigh, lateral part of the lower leg, dorsum of the foot and middle three toes, as well as the heel and plantar surface of the middle toes. The S1 dermatome extends from the buttock down the posterior surface of thigh and calf, and tends laterally to end in the region of the lateral malleolus and little toe on both dorsal and plantar surfaces. Motor function may also be affected, especially dorsiflexion (L4, 5), plantar flexion (S1, 2) or eversion (S1). In L5/S1 disc protrusion, examination of the calf muscles may reveal wasting, and the ankle jerk may be diminished or even absent.
[E:838; H:84]

587 Any abnormality of the hip joint may manifest itself as a limp. The 'dipping' gait seen in cases of congenital dislocation of the hip is due to the head of the femur slipping out of the acetabulum, therefore not allowing normal action of the ipsilateral abductors. This in turn means that the contralateral side of the pelvis does not elevate as it would in the normal, and the person is obliged to swing the whole lower trunk upwards to allow the leg to follow through. It is this swinging of the pelvis and lowering of the trunk on the affected side which produces the characteristic limp.
[B:250; D:222; E:605; F:367]

588 The blood supply of the head of the femur is from three routes. First, from the circumflex femoral arteries ascending in the synovial retinaculum along the femoral neck; second, from nutrient arteries ascending from the shaft; and,

lastly, a small contribution along the ligament of the head (ligamentum teres) which is often a branch from the obturator artery. Because most of these arteries run upwards along the neck, and because the capsule and retinacular arteries join low down the neck, a fracture through the neck itself is likely to interrupt the blood supply. Subcapital fractures particularly are prone to avascular necrosis, as the artery of the ligament of the head is not sufficient to keep the bone alive. A fracture through the trochanters, however, barely has an effect on the blood supply to the head, as the circumflex femoral vessels enter proximal to the break.
[D:235; G:449; H:301]

589 Shortening of the fractured femur is due to the strength of the longitudinally lying muscles, especially the quadriceps and hamstrings, as well as the adductor group which pull the leg superomedially. Also, instead of rotating about an axis between hip and knee, the femur now rotates about the axis of its shaft. This means that the upper adductors and iliopsoas now rotate the femur laterally, instead of medially as before.
[D:237; H:302]

590 Pure extension of the hip is normally limited to some 15–30° by the iliofemoral ligament and iliopsoas tendon. The movement easily mistaken for extension is, in fact, a combination of extension, pelvic tilt, abduction and lateral rotation. In testing extension, therefore, it is important, first, to fix the pelvis and, second, to perform the movement with the knee flexed. The hamstrings and gluteus maximus produce extension.
[D:242; E:518; G:442; H:300]

B Information answers

591 The femoral triangle is situated on the upper medial aspect of the front of the thigh. Its boundaries are the inguinal ligament superiorly, the sartorius laterally and the medial border of the adductor longus muscle medially. Its floor is composed, therefore, of adductor longus, pectineus and iliopsoas (from medial to

lateral). Its roof is the fascial layers and the skin of the thigh. It contains laterally the femoral nerve, splitting into its terminal branches, and medially a funnel-shaped fascial structure, the femoral sheath. This structure contains, from lateral to medial, the femoral artery, femoral vein and femoral canal which is full of fat and lymphatics. The lymphatics of the deep inguinal group are also situated in the femoral triangle.
[A:674, 676, 1053; C:392; G:420]

592 The quadriceps femoris is composed of four muscles, as its name suggests. They are all inserted into the patella and thence via the ligamentum patellae into the tuberosity of the tibia. Thus their combined action is to extend the knee. They are supplied by the femoral nerve.

The four heads are rectus femoris, vastus medialis, vastus intermedius and vastus lateralis. They arise from the femur, except rectus femoris which arises from the innominate bone via a straight head from the anterior inferior iliac spine and a reflected head from above the acetabulum. Therefore rectus femoris also has an action on the hip joint, which it flexes. Rectus femoris is a bipennate muscle situated anterior to the other three. Vastus intermedius arises from the front and the sides of the shaft of the femur, leaving only the medial and lateral lips of the linea aspera as origins for the vastus medialis and lateralis from which they respectively arise. The lowest fibres of vastus medialis are inserted into the medial aspect of the patella and run almost horizontally to this insertion, pulling the patella medially as they contract. This is because the 'carrying angle' between femur and tibia tends to make the pull of quadriceps lateral as well as upward. Without the medial pull of these medialis fibres, this contraction would tend to result in lateral dislocation of the patella.
[A:562; C:393; G:428]

593 The obturator nerve supplies the adductor group of muscles. These are five in number: adductor longus, adductor brevis, adductor magnus, gracilis and obturator externus. As

their name suggests, their principal function is to adduct the hip joint.

In general, they arise from the inferior ramus of the pubis and fan out to be inserted into the linea aspera. Gracilis, however, is inserted onto the upper medial aspect of the tibia and flexes the knee in addition to adducting the hip. Adductor magnus is really two muscles fused. It consists of an adductor portion, running from the pubis to linea aspera, supplied by the obturator nerve, and a hamstring portion running from the ischial tuberosity to the adductor tubercle on the femur. The latter is supplied by the tibial division of the sciatic nerve and extends the hip like all hamstrings.

Obturator externus arises from the outer aspect of the obturator membrane and adjacent pubis and ischium. Its tendon is inserted into the trochanteric fossa of the femur (a pit on the medial aspect of the greater trochanter). It rotates the hip laterally.
[A:564, 1052; C:400; G:425]

594 The adductor canal contains the femoral vessels, the terminal part of the obturator nerve, the saphenous nerve and the nerve to vastus medialis (both from the femoral nerve). It conducts them from the apex of the femoral triangle superiorly, to the adductor hiatus in adductor magnus inferiorly. It is a triangular cleft between muscles and has medial, anterior and posterior walls which are formed from sartorius, vastus medialis and adductor longus, respectively, in the upper part. Inferiorly, adductor magnus forms the posterior wall.
[A:674; C:395; E:512; G:425]

B Applied answers

595 A finger in the femoral canal will be in close contact with the femoral vein laterally, the lacunar ligament and conjoint tendon medially and the inguinal ligament (Poupart) and spermatic cord anteriorly. Posteriorly and deep to the femoral canal lies the superior ramus of the pubis and pectineus muscle. Due to these relationships, operations for enlarging the femoral canal or ring must be made medially or anteriorly.
[D:256; E:514; G:446; H:296]

596 To find the femoral vein it is most useful to know that it lies medial and parallel to the femoral artery, just below the inguinal ligament. The femoral artery is easily located by finding its pulsation mid-way between the anterior superior iliac spine and the pubic symphysis. Both artery and vein lie within the femoral sheath, so the vein tends to be well anchored. With one finger on the arterial pulsation, the needle is introduced 0.5 cm medially. It is not uncommon to sample venous blood mistakenly for arterial blood, as the two vessels are so close together.
[D:257; E:512; H:296]

597 A saphena varix is a swelling of the terminal part of the long saphenous vein near the cribriform fascia, which it pierces to join the femoral vein. This lies some 3–4 cm below and lateral to the pubic tubercle, and may even be mistaken for a femoral hernia as both may increase in size on coughing.
[C:362; H:297]

598 By observation, a femoral hernia lies below and lateral to the pubic tubercle, whereas an indirect inguinal hernia lies above the tubercle and passes either over or just medial to it.
[D:257; E:607]

599 The long saphenous vein is homologous to the cephalic vein, as are the short saphenous and basilic veins.
[G:49, 64]

600 The lymphatic drainage from the glans penis is to the superficial inguinal lymph nodes. This must not be confused with the lymphatic drainage of the testes, which is to the para-aortic nodes of the posterior abdominal wall.
[G:414; H:246]

601 A swelling within the psoas major muscle may cause pressure on parts of the lumbosacral nerve plexus which is found within its bulk. It is also possible that a swollen psoas muscle might compress structures passing below the inguinal ligament, such as the femoral nerve and its branches. The tingling in the big toe can be easily explained by pressure on the L4 spinal

nerve or the saphenous nerve (L4), which is the terminal sensory branch of the femoral nerve. The numbness on the lateral part of the buttock and thigh is due to compression of the lateral cutaneous nerve of the thigh as it passes below the inguinal ligament, just inferior to the anterior superior iliac spine.
[D:160; H:246, 250]

602 The long saphenous vein lies just anterior to the medial malleous at the ankle, and crosses the subcutaneous tibia or shinbone in the lower leg. It is here that the saphenous nerve often entwines round the vein, so during the operation to strip out the vein a portion of the nerve may easily be damaged.
[G:49; J:210]

603 Not only will the femoral artery and vein be endangered as they pass down the front of the thigh towards the subsartorial canal, but also their branches and tributaries. Mid-way down the thigh, a knife piercing sartorius and the femoral vessels will also lacerate adductor longus, a fairly thin muscle, and damage the profunda femoris vessels on its deep surface. The injury is therefore very bloody due to damage to two large arteries and their accompanying veins.
[E:518; H:298; J:192]

C Information answers

604 There are about a dozen bursae in the region of the knee joint. Three communicate with the joint: the suprapatellar bursa, the popliteus bursa and the medial gastrocnemius bursa. The suprapatellar (quadriceps) bursa extends one hand's breadth above the patella. Three further bursae are associated with the patella: the prepatellar bursa anterior to the bone, and the superficial and deep infrapatellar bursae on the respective sides of the ligamentum patellae. Other bursae are found around semimembranosus (between semimembranosus and the medial head of gastrocnemius) and around the collateral ligaments (one between the two parts of the tibial collateral ligament, one between the tibial collateral ligament and the pes anserinus,

and one between the fibular ligament and biceps). Other bursae have been described.
[A:455; H:310; F:375]

605 The cruciate ligaments are two intracapsular ligaments situated in the knee joint. They cross each other at right angles, hence their name. They derive their name from their tibial attachments. Thus the anterior cruciate ligament is attached to the anterior intercondylar area of the tibia. It passes upwards, backwards and laterally, to be attached to the medial aspect of the lateral femoral condyle. The posterior ligament is attached to the posterior tibial intercondylar area. It passes upwards, forwards and medially to the lateral aspect of the medial femoral condyle. The ligaments prevent anterior and posterior displacement of the tibia on the femur, the anterior ligament preventing anterior movement, the posterior ligament posterior displacement.

In extension the anterior ligament becomes taut. Further extension results in medial rotation of the femur on the tibia, causing all ligaments to tauten (including the posterior fibres of the posterior ligament) and locking of the knee. The anterior fibres of the posterior ligament become taut in flexion.
[A:454; C:459; F:367; G:458]

606 The menisci are formed from fibrocartilage and are situated between the femoral and tibial condyles, there being a medial and a lateral one in each knee joint. In cross-section they are triangular in shape, and thus deepen the tibial articulation for the femoral condyles. The medial meniscus is 'new moon'-shaped, its horns being attached to the intercondylar areas of the tibia. The convexity is tightly attached to the capsule and medial collateral ligament. Owing to this attachment, it is therefore the most commonly injured. The lateral meniscus is nearly circular and is deficient centrally. The popliteus tendon separates it from the capsule. It is therefore more mobile than the medial and less frequently injured. In hyperextension of the knee (locking) the tightening of the ligaments causes the menisci to become compressed.
[A:454; C:459; F:367; G:456]

607 The hamstrings consist of the semitendinosus, semimembranosus, the long head of biceps femoris and half of adductor magnus. They all arise from the ischial tuberosity, are supplied by the tibial division of the sciatic nerve and are situated on the posterior aspect of the thigh. With the exception of adductor magnus, they are inserted into the upper aspect of the lower leg bones. Semitendinosus is inserted into the upper part of the subcutaneous surface of the tibia behind sartorius and gracilis. Semimembranosus is inserted via a broad aponeurosis to the posterior aspect of the medial tibial condyle, the posterior part of the knee joint capsule forming the oblique popliteal ligament, and over popliteus to the soleal line. Biceps is inserted into the head of the fibula. Together, the hamstrings flex the knee and extend the hip.

Adductor magnus reaches only as far inferiorly as the adductor tubercle of the femur. It cannot therefore have an action on the knee.
[A:570; C:410; E:522; G:431]

608 The knee jerk involves stretching the ligamentum patellae by striking it with a hammer. This in turn stretches the muscle fibres of the quadriceps femoris group (rectus femoris, vastus medialis, vastus intermedius, vastus lateralis). The stretch receptors in the muscles thus excited send sensory impulses to the spinal cord via the femoral nerve (L2, 3, 4). Motor impulses are sent back to the quadriceps via the same nerve, causing the muscles to contract. The knee jerk depends on the integrity of the quadriceps muscle and ligamentum patellae, both sensory and motor limbs of the femoral nerve and the spinal cord in segments L2, 3 and 4.
[A:753, 800, 826; B:28; C:67]

609 The popliteal fossa is situated behind the knee joint. Its floor may be divided into thirds. From superior to inferior, this is formed by the popliteal surface of the femur, the capsule of the knee joint and the fascia covering popliteus. Its roof is the skin and superficial and deep fasciae of this portion of the lower limb. Its boundaries are: laterally, biceps femoris and the lateral head of gastrocnemius (from top to bottom); medially, semimembranosus and semitendinosus above and the medial head of gastroc-

nemius below. It contains connective tissue, lymph nodes, the popliteal artery and vein, and the terminal branches of the sciatic nerve. The popliteal artery is the continuation of the femoral artery as it passes through the adductor hiatus. It is the deepest structure in the popliteal fossa. It is accompanied by the popliteal vein. The short saphenous vein pierces the deep fascia of the fossa to enter the popliteal vein. The sciatic nerve bifurcates under biceps into the common peroneal and tibial nerves. The former runs along biceps across the lateral aspect of the fossa. The latter runs superficial to the popliteal vessels in the fossa's median plane.
[A:678; E:538; G:451]

610 Popliteus arises by muscular fibres from the upper medial aspect of the tibia above the soleal line. It passes upwards and laterally, to be inserted via a tendon into a depression just below the lateral epicondyle of the femur. The tendon lies within the capsule of the knee. The popliteus medially rotates the tibia on the femur. During extension, the ligaments of the knee become taut by lateral rotation of the tibia on the femur. This 'locks' the knee. For flexion to occur, 'unlocking' must first take place. This action is performed by popliteus, which medially rotates the tibia on the femur.
[A:576; C:454; E:554]

C Applied answers

611 Pains in the knee may in fact be due to referred pain from the hip joint. The nerve supply of the hip joint is usually from the femoral nerve and branches from the obturator, with occasional contributions from the nerve to quadratus femoris and the superior gluteal nerve. The knee has a very similar supply, with the femoral, obturator and sciatic nerves all contributing some twigs to the joint. It is easy to see how pain from the two joints is easily confused by the brain. In general, the nerves which cross a joint give branches to that joint (Hilton's law).
[D:244]

612 The medial meniscus or semilunar cartilage is most commonly torn because it is attached

directly to the medial collateral ligament. When a twisting injury affects the knee joint, tension is applied to the collateral ligaments. If the meniscus is held taut by the medial ligament and the bony condyles continue to move, then a tear may appear in the meniscus. 'Bucket handle' tears of the medial meniscus are quite common and are usually felt as pain along the joint line itself.
[G:461; H:309; J:276]

613 In extension, the patella is anterior to the knee joint and femur, but is separated from them by the synovial membrane and suprapatellar bursa. A knee joint distended with an effusion results in fluid lying in this intervening space, and when pressed down sharply the patella can be bounced up and down on this fluid cushion. The fluid often tracks to the suprapatellar pouch, or bursa, deep to the quadriceps tendon, and may lie some 5 cm superior to the patella.
[G:468; H:310]

614 Swellings of the bursae around the knee are named after certain occupations which are supposed to cause trauma, and hence effusions, of these bursae. Housemaid's knee is a swelling of the prepatellar bursa, which lies anterior to the lower part of the patella and upper ligamentum patellae. This swelling is said to be caused by scrubbing floors on hands and knees. Clergyman's knee is said to be due to excessive kneeling at prayer! It is an effusion in one of the infrapatellar bursae which lie between the tibia and ligamentum patellae and the skin.
[G:468; H:310]

615 The patella is the largest sesamoid bone and ossifies around the age of 3 years. Women dislocate their patellae more commonly than men, probably due to their wider pelvis and therefore increased lateral pull of the quadriceps. Factors which prevent lateral patellar dislocation include the horizontal direction of the lower fibres of vastus medialis, the size and height of the lateral femoral condyle and the shape of the patella itself. The last two features are readily seen on a skyline view x-ray of the knee.
[C:387; F:369; H:278]

616 The patella is a sesamoid bone which develops in hyaline cartilage, and begins to ossify from several centres at about 3 years. The supero-lateral angle may ossify independently. These congenital bipartite patellae are easily confused with a fracture.
[C:387; H:278]

617 The ossification centres of the distal end of the femur and proximal end of the tibia are used in determining a baby's age. The centre of ossifica-tion for the distal end of the femur usually appears before birth, in both sexes, whereas the proximal tibial centre appears at birth. The presence or absence of these two epiphyses on an x-ray can give a fairly good idea of the age of the baby at the time of death.
[C:434; G:291]

618 A torn meniscus, which is more commonly the medial, may result in a loose segment of the cartilage moving independently within the joint. This free-moving cartilage may become wedged between the articular surfaces of tibia and femur, making further extension imposs-ible and thus 'locking' the knee. A minor form of this condition may cause a 'clicking' knee joint.
[E:573; G:457; H:309]

619 The popliteal pulse is extremely difficult to palpate in most people. This is because it is the deepest-lying structure in the popliteal fossa. Having pierced the adductor magnus at the adductor hiatus, it lies anterior to its vein and the tibial nerve in the popliteal fossa. All these structures are embedded in fat, and both the artery and the vein are additionally surrounded by a tough fibrous sheath. Flexion of the knee often facilitates palpation due to relaxation of nerve and sheath.
[E:540; G:454; H:306]

620 All the structures passing through the popliteal fossa may cause a swelling in this region. A popliteal aneurysm and popliteal or short sa-phenous varicosities are the most likely causes. However, neuromata of the tibial, sural or com-mon peroneal nerves can occur as well as effu-sions in the semimembranosus bursae, or a

cystic swelling originating from the joint capsule itself (Baker's cyst).
[E:540; G:453; H:307]

621 The three tendons most easily palpable, often visible at the back of the knee in flexion, are biceps femoris laterally, and semitendinosus and semimembranosus medially.
[C:388; H:304]

622 This is a typical 'bumper-bar' injury which usually results in at least a fractured neck of the fibula. At this site, the common peroneal nerve winds into the lateral, and later the anterior, compartment of the lower leg, and so is often damaged. The branches of the common peroneal nerve are the superficial and deep peroneal nerves. The deep nerve runs with the anterior tibial artery to supply the extensor group of muscles including tibialis anterior, whereas the superficial peroneal nerve gives muscular branches to the peronei muscles which are the major evertors of the foot. Damage to the deep peroneal nerve results, therefore, in an inability to dorsiflex the foot, whilst an injured superficial peroneal nerve results in an inverted foot. A combination of these is 'foot-drop' which is thus seen as an inverted plantar flexed foot. This results in the patient catching his big toe on the swing-through and scuffing the anterolateral part of his shoes when he walks.
[G:453; H:305]

D Information answers

623 The interosseous membrane running between fibula and tibia separates the leg into an anterior (extensor) compartment and a posterior (flexor) compartment. The peroneal muscles attached to lateral aspect of the fibula form a third, lateral, compartment. Each compartment is served by its own nerve—viz. anterior: deep peroneal nerve; posterior: tibial nerve; lateral: superficial peroneal nerve. The anterior compartment consists of tibialis anterior, extensor hallucis longus, extensor digitorum longus and peroneus tertius. The posterior compartment may be subdivided into superficial and deep parts. The superficial part comprises gastrocne-

mius, plantaris and soleus. The deep part consists of popliteus, flexor digitorum longus, flexor hallucis longus and tibialis posterior. The two parts are separated by a fascial septum—the deep transverse fascia of the leg. The lateral compartment contains peroneus longus and peroneus brevis.
[A:571; E:534; G:472]

624 The principal plantar flexors of the ankle are gastrocnemius and soleus, which insert onto the calcaneum. In theory, the muscles passing behind the flexor and peroneal retinacula should also be plantar flexors—viz. peroneus longus, peroneus brevis, tibialis posterior, flexor digitorum longus and flexor hallucis longus. Their mechanical advantage is poor, however, and cutting the tendo calcaneus results in severe weakness of this movement.

Dorsiflexion is performed by those muscles passing anterior to the joint; viz. tibialis anterior, extensor hallucis longus, extensor digitorum and peroneus tertius.
[A:571, 574; C:450; E:552; G:482]

625 The tissues of the lower limb, superficial to the deep fascia, are drained of venous blood by the great and small saphenous veins. Both arise from the venous network on the dorsum of the foot. The great saphenous vein arises from the medial aspect of this network. It ascends, passing immediately anterior to the medial malleolus. It continues upwards and backwards on the medial aspect of the leg, in company with the saphenous nerve, to pass a hand's breadth behind the medial side of the patella. It curves fowards as it ascends the thigh to reach the saphenous opening 2.5 cm below the inguinal ligament, where it pierces the deep fascia and enters the femoral vein. Various perforating veins run between the great saphenous vein and the deep veins of the calf. The small saphenous vein arises from the lateral aspect of the venous network of the dorsum of the foot. It ascends immediately behind the lateral malleolus and passes upwards and posteriorly to reach the middle of the back of the leg. It runs upwards in company with the sural nerve to the popliteal fossa, where it pierces the deep fascia and enters the popliteal vein.
[A:704; C:362; E:508; G:49]

626 At the ankle, each tendon is contained within a synovial sheath which lubricates it as it moves under a retinaculum which ties the tendon down and prevents 'bowstringing'. The inferior extensor retinaculum consists of superficial and deep layers. The tendons run between these layers in their synovial sheaths, separated from their neighbours by septa which join the superficial and deep parts. From medial to lateral, these extensor tendons are tibialis anterior, extensor hallucis longus, extensor digitorum longus and peroneus tertius.
[A:572, 578; C:439; G:479]

627 The peronei are so named because they take origin from the fibula (L. *fibula*, Gk. *peroneus* = skewer). Peroneus longus originates from the upper two-thirds of the fibula's lateral surface, peroneus brevis from the lower two-thirds. Both tendons run behind the lateral malleolus and are held in position by the peroneal retinaculum. The tendons are separated by the peroneal tubercle of the calcaneum—the brevis passing above it, the longus below, and both being held in position by the inferior peroneal retinaculum. Peroneus brevis is inserted into the base of the fifth metatarsal. Peroneus longus enters a groove in the cuboid and crosses deep in the sole of the foot, to be inserted into the base of the first metatarsal and adjacent medial cuneiform. Both are supplied by the superficial branch of the common peroneal nerve. Both muscles plantar flex the ankle. They are also evertors, the movement occurring at the tarsal joints. This is their unique action, no other muscle being capable of this. Peroneus longus helps support the transverse arch of the foot as it crosses the sole. Peroneus brevis maintains the lateral longitudinal arch.
[A:573, 1060; E:548; F:342]

628 Around the ankle joint the deep fascia is thickened in various regions to form a series of retinacula which bind the tendons down and keep them in position. The extensor tendons are held in place by two extensor retinacula—superior and inferior. The superior is attached to the anterior aspects of the tibia and fibula. It is split to enclose tibialis anterior. The inferior extensor retinaculum is the shape of a Y lying

on its side. The base is attached to the upper anterior aspect of the calcaneum. The superior limb is attached to the medial malleolus, the inferior to the plantar fascia. The tendons of tibialis anterior, extensor hallucis longus, extensor digitorum and peroneus tertius are held in place by the extensor retinaculum. The anterior tibial vessels and deep peroneal nerve also run under it. The flexor retinaculum extends from the medial malleolus to the medial aspect of the calcaneum. Tibialis posterior, flexor digitorum longus, flexor hallucis longus, the posterior tibial vessels and tibial nerve run deep to this structure. The peroneal muscles are held in place by two peroneal retinacula—superior and inferior. The superior encompasses both the longus and brevis tendons and runs from the lateral malleolus to the calcaneum. The inferior retinaculum is attached to the peroneal tubercle of the calcaneum, which separates the two tendons (brevis being superior). It is attached above and below to the calcaneum.
[A:578; C:439; E:556]

629 The ankle joint is a synovial joint of the hinge variety. Being a hinge, it has strong collateral ligaments to prevent movements other than in the anteroposterior plane. The medial ligament (deltoid ligament) is triangular. Its apex is attached to the medial malleolus. Its base consists of a superficial and a deep part. The deep fibres are attached to the talus, the superficial fibres to the navicular (anteriorly), calcaneum (centrally) and talus (posteriorly). The lateral ligament consists of three distinct parts: the anterior talofibular ligament (anteriorly), running from lateral malleolus to the lateral surface of the talus; the calcaneofibular ligament (centrally), running from lateral malleolus to calcaneum; and the posterior talofibular ligament (posteriorly), running from the medial aspect of the lateral malleolus to the posterior tubercle of the talus.
[A:460; C:477; E:576; F:378; G:4115]

630 The ankle jerk is elicited by tapping the tendo calcaneus (Achilles) with a hammer. This stretches the muscles attached to it (i.e. gastrocnemius and soleus). Afferent impulses pass via sensory fibres in the tibial nerve, which sup-

plies these muscles, to cord segments L5, S1 and 2. Efferent impulses travel from these segments via motor fibres in the tibial nerve to these same muscles, causing them to contract. The presence of the ankle jerk depends therefore upon the integrity of the gastrocnemius and soleus, the tendo calcaneus, the sensory and motor limbs of the tibial nerve, and cord segments L5, S1 and 2.
[A:753, 801, 1056; C:67; E:37]

D Applied answers

631 Gastrocnemius originates from the femoral condyles, whereas soleus originates from the fibula and soleal line of the tibia and does not cross the knee joint. Both insert together as the tendo calcaneus. In order to demonstrate them separately, one must first flex the knee to neutralise gastrocnemius and then resist plantar flexion. This will single out soleus, whereas with the knee extended both will contract in plantar flexion.
[E:540; G:454; H:315]

632 The short saphenous vein and branches of the sural nerve may be in very close contact on the calf, so stripping out the vein may traumatise the sural nerve, which supplies the skin of the lateral side of the foot and little toe. For the same reason, stripping the long saphenous vein may leave tingling in the big toe due to damage to the saphenous nerve.
[B:200; C:363; H:317]

633 In most cases it is the deep venous system which is investigated. This is achieved by injection of contrast medium into a superficial vein on the dorsum of the foot, and constricture bands are placed at the ankle and below the knee. Occlusion of the superficial veins causes the deep venous system to fill. Indications for this procedure include diagnosis of deep vein thrombosis, and the location of varicosities in the perforating veins which pass from superficial to deep venous systems.
[B:202; J:210]

634 The most constant site of the long saphenous vein which, prior to the popularisation of central venous catheterisation, was commonly used for 'cut-downs', is at the ankle. Here the vein runs 2–3 cm anterior to the medial malleolus, and can be seen or palpated in most normal individuals.
[F:310; H:318]

635 The tendo calcaneus is the strongest tendon in the body and ruptures only if violent force is used. Usually this happens to athletes or entertainers who carry on their sport beyond their prime, though the popularity of such sports as squash and rock climbing has produced quite a few young people with this injury. The foot is useless, as any active plantar flexion proves impossible. Many surgeons advise operative suture as early as possible.
[E:552; G:478; H:321]

636 Normally, most people have both a posterior tibial pulse (felt just behind the tendon of flexor digitorum longus at the medial malleolus) and a dorsalis pedis pulse (felt on the dorsum of the foot between the tendons of extensor hallucis longus and extensor digitorum longus). Usually the dorsalis pedis artery is a direct continuation of the anterior tibial artery, but occasionally the arterial supply of the foot is from a perforating branch of the peroneal artery and in these cases the dorsalis pedis pulsation is very weak or even absent. Absence of either posterior tibial or dorsalis pedis pulsation occurs in about 5 per cent of the normal population.
[G:477; H:318]

637 The ankle joint is most unstable with the foot plantar flexed, which happens when one is standing on one's toes or walking downstairs. However, in dorsiflexion it is a rigid stable joint. This is due to the shape of the talus, which is broader anteriorly. In dorsiflexion the talus is forced into the tibiofibular socket, pushing these bones slightly apart and causing the malleoli to grip the talus firmly, producing a very firm platform.
[B:244; F:351; H:323]

638 A torn deltoid (medial) ligament is a serious injury for two reasons. First, it causes instability

248

of the ankle joint because this ligament maintains the mortise effect of the tibia and fibula with the talus, by connecting the medial malleolus to the sustentaculum tali and tuberosity of the navicular bone. Second, it attaches to the plantar calcaneonavicular ligament (spring), which is most important in maintaining the medial longitudinal arch of the foot.
[E:577; G:4115; H:323]

639 In 1768, Percival Pott described a lateral outward fracture-dislocation of the ankle. This injury has retained his name, and is divided into three degrees of severity. The first degree involves a fracture of the lateral malleolus alone, the fracture line running obliquely upwards and backwards. The second degree involves the talus moving laterally, causing an oblique lateral malleolar fracture with either a transverse fracture of the medial malleolus or severe disruption of the deltoid ligament. The third degree cases are due to continued rotational forces on the talus, forcing it laterally and backwards. This produces fractures of both malleoli and of the posterior portion of the tibial articular surface. A third degree fracture thus leaves a most unstable ankle, often with three separate fracture lines. Internal fixation with pins is required to maintain the original position of the mortise joint into which the talus fits.
[D:251; J:88]

E Information answers

640 Two types of muscle fibre may be recognised in some animals—red and white. The red fibres contain more myoglobin, hence the colour, and have more abundant granular sarcoplasm. White muscle is capable of sudden rapid contraction, as in movement of a joint. Red muscle is able to contract in a more leisurely and sustained manner and is important for the maintenance of posture. In chickens the distinction between red muscle, in the legs, and white muscle in the breast, is obvious, but in man all muscle contains both types of fibre, though in different proportions. Thus gastroc-

nemius has a higher proportion of white fibres, and soleus a higher number of red.
[A:480; F:22]

641　The four named nerves which supply sensation to the dorsum of the foot are the saphenous nerve, the sural nerve, the deep peroneal nerve and the superficial peroneal nerve. The saphenous nerve—a branch of the femoral nerve—supplies skin on the medial side of the leg and the adjacent area of the dorsum of the foot as far as the metatarsophalangeal joint of the hallux. The sural nerve—a branch of the tibial nerve—runs behind the lateral malleolus onto the lateral side of the foot, supplying it on dorsal and plantar aspects. It also supplies the little toe. The deep peroneal nerve supplies, via its medial terminal branch, a wedge of skin on the dorsum of the foot on adjacent sides of the hallux and second toes. The remainder of the dorsum is supplied by the superficial peroneal nerve via its medial and lateral terminal branches.
[A:1056; E:569; G:47]

642　Inversion is the movement which makes the sole face medially. It is performed by muscles which pass on the medial side of the ankle; viz. tibialis anterior and tibialis posterior. Eversion results in the sole facing laterally. It is performed by peroneus longus and brevis which pass lateral to the ankle. The movement occurs at the joints below the ankle—the transverse tarsal and mid-tarsal joints.
[A:464; F:379]

643　The arches of the foot are the medial and lateral longitudinal arches and the transverse arch. The last is only a half-arch, being deficient medially. Various factors are involved in their maintenance. First, the bones are wedge-shaped, tapering inferiorly. Second, the bones are bound together by ligaments. The ligaments on the plantar aspect are the stronger. Third, the ends of the arches are connected by muscles and tendons like a bowstring. Fourth, the arches are suspended from above by long tendons; viz. peroneus longus, tibialis posterior and tibialis anterior. The medial longitudinal arch consists of calcaneum, talus, navicular, medial cuneiform and first metatarsal. The in-

ferior aspects of these bones are connected by the calcaneonavicular ligament. The plantar aponeurosis, flexor hallucis longus, abductor hallucis and the medial portion of the flexor digitorum muscles connect the two ends of the arch. Tibialis anterior and posterior suspend the navicular from above. The lateral arch consists of calcaneum, cuboid and fifth metatarsal. They are tied together by long and short plantar ligaments inferiorly. The ends of the arch are joined by the plantar aponeurosis, abductor digiti minimi and the lateral portion of the flexor digitorum muscles. The peroneal muscles suspend it from above. The transverse arch is between the cuneiform (wedge-shaped) bones and the metatarsal bases, held together by the deep transverse plantar and interosseus ligaments, and suspended by peroneus longus and tibialis posterior.
[A:469; E:581; F:382]

644 The line of gravity passes through the body of the axis, anterior to the thoracic spine and sacrum. It then passes behind the hip joints but anterior to the knee and ankle joints.
[A:584; B:249; F:15]

645 In walking, one lower limb supports the body weight while the other is swinging forwards. The roles of supporting and swinging are then reversed.

Let us consider the right leg to be swinging and the left leg to be supporting initially. As the right foot is taken off the ground the pelvis is tilted by the left abductors (gluteus medius and minimus), so that the right ilium is raised. This allows the foot to clear the ground during swinging. The right hip flexes, swinging the right leg forwards, first by gravity and then by iliopsoas. The right knee is also flexed, by gravity and the hamstrings, and the foot is dorsiflexed by the extensors and tibialis anterior. This flexion of the knee and extension of the ankle further increase the clearance of the limb from the ground during the swinging phase. As the limb is moved anterior to the axis of the body, the knee is extended by the quadriceps. The right ilium is thrust forwards and the right leg rotated laterally to keep it in line with the direction of movement. The ankle is plantar-flexed as the foot approaches the ground. As the right foot touches the ground, the supporting phase commences. The left hip abductors are relaxed and the pelvis returns to its level attitude. The body weight is moved anteriorly from the heel along the outer side of the sole of the foot to the metatarsal heads. At the same time, the body weight is brought above the right foot by extension of the hip (gluteus maximus and hamstrings). The knee is kept extended and the foot dorsiflexes as the body moves over it.

As the body weight moves anterior to the position of the right foot, the foot is plantar-flexed (gastrocnemius and soleus) and the heel leaves the ground. The metatarsophalangeal joints are flexed as a consequence. The flexor muscles of the toes (particularly flexor hallucis longus) now contract and push the body weight forwards to take the next step. The right foot leaves the ground and the process is repeated. [A:584; B:250; C:486]

646 Lymph from the superficial tissues of the heel will run in the lymphatics following one or other of the saphenous veins. That following the great saphenous vein will eventually drain to the vertically disposed groups of superficial inguinal nodes around the termination of the vein. The lymph vessels following the small saphenous vein will pierce the deep fascia in the popliteal fossa and enter the popliteal nodes. From here lymph passes to the deep inguinal nodes around the femoral vein in the femoral triangle.
[A:735; C:364; E:525; I:197]

E Applied answers

647 In severe inversion injuries, tension is exerted on the laterally placed muscles and, in particular, the peronei. Peroneus brevis, originating from the fibula, inserts into the tuberosity of the fifth metatarsal. Tension on this insertion often results in its fracture. However, a fracture should not be confused with an epiphysis, which is frequently present at this site.
[D:251; E:577; G:478; H:321]

648 Talipes equinovarus is a deformity of the foot, consisting of the hindfoot being drawn up by a tight tendo calcaneus (L. *equino* = horse-like) the sole facing inwards (varus), as well as a slight adduction of the forefoot. The head of the talus may be felt anterior to the lateral malleolus, instead of in its normal position below and anterior to the medial malleolus. This new position allows the anterior compartment (tibial) muscles to draw the foot into further adduction. It may be a congenital deformity, for which intrauterine pressure has been blamed, or it may be found secondarily to conditions such as spina bifida.
[B:248; C:434]

649 Pes planus is true flattening of the longitudinal arch, caused by abnormalities of the talonavicular joint, naviculocuneiform joint or cuneiform–first metatarsal joints. These may be of bony origin or of muscular origin, the latter being due to inefficiency of the tibialis posterior tendon in maintaining the arch.
[B:248; C:434; H:323]

650 Pes cavus is an abnormal elevation of the longitudinal arch, which is seen in numerous neurological disorders such as poliomyelitis, spina bifida or Friedreich's ataxia. It is due to shortening of the plantar muscles and fascia. In severe cases, lack of the interossei muscles may result in severe clawing which eventually leads to dorsal subluxation at the metatarsophalangeal joints. Occasionally, an extremely high arch may require removal of a bony wedge from the talus for its correction.
[B:248; C:434; G:411; H:323]

651 Lumbar sympathectomy will remove the sympathetic outflow to the arteries of the lower limb, and thus cause dilatation of the collateral circulation in a leg with occlusive arterial disease of the main vessels. This operation is also sometimes carried out to benefit patients with chronic severe chilblains, by increasing the blood flow to the cold, blotchy feet. It is similar in rationale to thoracocervical sympathectomy for Raynaud's disease of the hands.
[C:668; D:165; G:2119; H:242]

BACK

A Information answers

652 A typical cervical vertebra is slender in structure. Its body is wider from side to side than
anteroposteriorly and possesses small synovial
joints laterally. It has a large triangular vertebral
foramen and small spines which are bifid. The
transverse process has a hole in it, the foramen
transversarium, for the vertebral vessels. No
other vertebra possesses these structures.

   The thoracic vertebra possesses two facets on
each side of the body, and one on its transverse
process for the articulation of the ribs. No other
vertebra has these facets. Its body is heart-
shaped and the long spines slope inferiorly. The
articular facets are in the vertical plane.

   The lumbar vertebrae are relatively much
more massive, with a large kidney-shaped
body. The spines are quadrangular in shape
and face directly backwards. The articular facets
are arranged in the sagittal plane.
[A:233; D:344; E:814]

653 The spinous process of the seventh cervical
vertebra is the most easily palpated, being
much longer than the others. For this reason it
is called the vertebra prominens.
[A:236; E:812]

654 During development the body of a vertebra is
formed from a central mass—the centrum—and
the two lateral parts of the neural arch. The
centrum of the atlas is fused to the centrum of
the axis, forming the dens (odontoid peg). The
atlas is therefore missing the bulk of its body.
[A:235; E:766]

655 The iliac crests lie on a transverse plane through
the level of the fourth lumbar vertebra. This is
the level of the bifurcation of the abdominal
aorta. Clinically, this plane is commonly used
as a surface marking for lumbar punctures.
[A:346; D:58]

656 The direction of movement allowed between
adjacent vertebrae depends upon the shape and
direction of the articular processes. In the lum-

bar region the sagittal disposition of these allows flexion and extension more readily than other movements.
[A:413; E:817; H:76]

657 Vertebral bodies are joined by secondary cartilaginous joints. Each vertebral body is covered at its articular end with hyaline cartilage. Between the hyaline cartilage covering adjacent vertebral bodies is a fibrocartilaginous disc. These joints are strengthened by the anterior and posterior longitudinal ligaments.

Between the lateral aspects of the bodies of adjacent cervical vertebrae there are in addition to the secondary cartilaginous joints, on each side a small synovial joint (neurocentral joints).
[A:411; E:820; G:519]

658 The specialised ligaments of the atlantoaxial joint are the transverse ligament of the atlas and the two alar ligaments.

The transverse ligament of the atlas unites the lateral masses of the atlas and runs posterior to the dens of the axis. It holds the dens firmly against the anterior arch of the atlas like a strap, preventing its posterior displacement towards the spinal cord but allowing rotation.

The alar ligaments, one on each side, arise from the top of the dens and run superolaterally to the medial sides of the occipital condyles. They hold the skull to the atlantoaxial unit, and limit rotation of the atlantoaxial joint.
[A:415; G:539]

659 The ligamentum nuchae is found in the cervical region, and is the continuation of the interspinous and supraspinous ligaments of the thoracic and lumbar vertebrae. It is attached to the external occipital crest and spines of the cervical vertebrae.

In quadrupedal mammals with large protuberant necks (e.g. horses) it is well developed, contains abundant elastic tissue and helps support the head. Man stands vertically, supporting his head on the cervical vertebrae, and consequently the human ligamentum nuchae is poorly developed.
[A:413; E:818]

660 The bodies of the vertebrae are united by the anterior and posterior longitudinal ligaments.

The anterior longitudinal ligament is attached to the anterior surfaces of the bodies and intervertebral discs. The posterior longitudinal ligament lies in the vertebral canal and is attached to the posterior surfaces of the discs and margins of the bodies but not to the central portion of the bodies.

The spines are joined by interspinous ligaments, which run between adjacent spines, and the supraspinous ligaments, which are attached to the tips of the spinous processes.
[A:411; E:818]

661 The ligamenta flava join the laminae of adjacent vertebrae and with them form the posterior wall of the vertebral canal. They contain an abundance of yellow elastic tissue, hence their name (L. *flavus* = yellow).
[A:413; D:349; H:86]

A Applied answers

662 Kyphosis is a hump back (Gk. *kyphos* = humpbacked) and is used to describe an abnormal spinal curvature with a backward convexity. Scoliosis comes from the Greek for crookedness, and is a lateral curvature of the spine. Lordosis is a hollow back, and a degree of lumbar lordosis is found in all normal healthy people.
[E:837]

663 Spina bifida is a failure of closure of the neural groove with associated abnormalities of the related mesoderm, resulting in an incomplete bony neural arch. Most often found in the lumbosacral region, this condition is fairly common, especially in Wales and north-west England, and although no specific biochemical or chromosomal defect has been identified, it certainly has a familial tendency. Cytoplasmic inheritance has been suggested to explain the frequency amongst siblings. Different degrees of spina bifida range from complete non-fusion, myelocele through meningomyelocele, meningocele, to spina bifida occulta, where only the bony canal is abnormal. This may be suggested by a thick tuft of hair in the lumbar region overlying the defect. These malformations of

the spinal cord may result in incontinence and paralysis of the lower limbs.
[A:111; C:322]

664 The posterior superior iliac spine is a most useful landmark for marrow punctures because, first, the patient does not watch the procedure and, second, a greater volume of marrow can be aspirated from this region than from other red-marrow-containing areas. The skin dimple above the buttock is the surface marking and the needle is inserted 1 cm below and laterally, i.e. in the plane of the innominate bone.
[B:546]

665 On viewing this x-ray, the outline resembling a small Scottish terrier can be seen. Its nose is the transverse process, the eye the pedicle, whilst the superior articular process forms the tip of the ear. The dog's neck is the 'pars interarticularis'—a radiological term equivalent to the anterior part of the lamina. Defects of ossification in the pars may lead to spondylolisthesis.
[I:560; J:106]

666 Cervical vertebrae are prone to dislocation due to the almost horizontal alignment of the articular facets.
[G:55; H:76]

667 Death. This sudden event may be caused by the fractured dens being driven into the spinal cord. This may be the cause of death when judicial hanging is carried out.
[B:543; H:83]

668 To find entry into the vertebral artery above the level of C6 requires more luck than judgement, as the artery then lies in the bony foramina transversaria until it enters the skull through the foramen magnum. Once inside the skull, it joins its fellow to become the basilar artery lying on the clivus. The vein, however, often stays inside the foramen of C7 unaccompanied by the artery.
[G:983; H:82]

669 A posterior prolapse of the C2/3 disc may cause pressure on the spinal cord above the phrenic

nerve outflow of C3, 4 and 5. If this happens suddenly, respiration will cease and, if not maintained artificially, the patient will die.
[C:311; E:817]

670　When performing a cisternal puncture, with the needle lying just under the occiput and the patient's neck flexed, the needle is advanced in a plane which passes through the external auditory meatus and the nasion. To enter the cisterna magna the needle must pass through the skin and superficial fascia and through the ligamentum nuchae which is the cranial extension of both the supraspinous and interspinous ligaments. Having pierced the posterior atlanto-occipital membrane, the continuation of the ligamenta flava, the tip lies amongst the posterior vertebral venous plexus of the epidural space. This lies at about 3 cm depth, and to enter the cisterna the needle must be advanced gently through the dura and arachnoid. It is worth remembering that the vertebral arteries lie only 1.5 cm lateral to the midline and that the medulla is just 1 cm or so in advance of the needle tip! Paediatric deaths or injury can happen during this procedure.
[H:66; I:391]

671　A prolapsed intervertebral disc is most commonly seen in the lower lumbar region at L4/5 or L5/S1. The consequences include low back pain and shooting pains down the leg towards the foot, often termed sciatica. On examination, the patient has great difficulty in performing the straight-leg test due to pain caused by stretching of the sciatic nerve.
[B:533; G:519]

B　Information questions

672　The erector spinae is better termed the sacrospinalis. It arises from the median sacral crest and ascends in the grooves on either side between the vertebral spines and their transverse processes. It splits in the lumbar region into three: a lateral group of muscles (iliocostalis), an intermediate group (longissimus) and a medial group (spinalis).
[A:511; C:327; G:527]

673　The transversospinalis group of muscles is composed of three groups. From superficial to deep, these are the semispinalis group (thoracis, cervicis, capitis), multifidus and the rotatores group (cervicis, thoracis and lumborum). These muscles run upwards and medially from the transverse processes of vertebrae to the vertebral spines. Those of semispinalis span about five interspaces, those of multifidus about three and rotatores one or two.
[A:512; H:88]

674　All the deep muscles of the back are supplied by the posterior primary rami of the spinal nerves.
[A:1032; E:815]

675　The dorsal ramus of C1 (suboccipital nerve) does not have any sensory territory, unlike other dorsal rami. The suboccipital nerve does, however, contain motor fibres and supplies the four muscles of the suboccipital triangle (superior oblique, inferior oblique, rectus capitis posterior major and rectus capitis posterior minor).
[A:514; G:534]

676　The ventral rami of C2 and 3 contribute to the sensory supply of the back of the neck via the greater auricular nerve (C2, 3) and the lesser occipital nerve (C2). The greater auricular nerve supplies skin over the parotid, mastoid process and posterior inferior aspect of the auricle. The lesser occipital nerve supplies skin over the upper posterior part of sternomastoid. The remainder of the back of the neck is supplied by the posterior rami of the spinal nerves.
[A:1036; E:626]

677　The small muscles of the suboccipital region are rectus capitis posterior major, rectus capitis posterior minor, inferior oblique and superior oblique. Their main action is to help stabilise the skull and cancel out the unwanted movements of the prime movers (sternomastoid, semispinalis, splenius, etc). They are all supplied by the posterior ramus of C1. Flexion and extension movements in this region occur at the altanto-occipital joint (nodding); rotation movements occur at the atlantoaxial joint (shaking). Rectus capitis posterior major runs from the occiput to C2 and thus acts over both joints.

It is the only muscle to do this, and it extends the head and rotates it to its own side. Rectus capitis posterior minor runs from the occiput to the posterior arch of the atlas. It extends the head. The inferior oblique runs from the spine of the axis to the lateral mass of the atlas. It rotates the skull and atlas to its own side. The superior oblique muscle runs from occiput to the lateral mass of the atlas. It is a lateral flexor of the skull on the atlas.
[A:513; G:535]

678 The most vital structure in the suboccipital triangle is the vertebral artery (third part). It exits the foramen transversarium of the atlas and curves backwards behind the lateral mass of the atlas to lie in a groove on the upper surface of the posterior arch of the atlas, and enters the foramen magnum. It is destined to supply the hindbrain—hence its importance.
[A:514; F:475; G:538]

679 The suboccipital triangle is bounded by the rectus capitis posterior major muscle, the superior oblique muscle and the inferior oblique muscle. Its roof is skin and dense fibrofatty tissue; below this, its floor is the lateral aspect of the posterior arch of the atlas and the posterior atlanto-occipital membrane.
[A:513; G:535]

B Applied answers

680 The auscultation triangle overlies the sixth intercostal space of the back and its boundaries are trapezius, latissimus dorsi and the rhomboid muscles, and it is a particularly good site to hear chest sounds due to its lack of covering muscle.

The lumbar triangle of Petit, whose floor is the internal oblique muscle, is bounded by latissimus dorsi, external oblique's free posterior border and the iliac crest. Rarely, it is the site of a lumbar hernia.
[G:2122; H:87, 111]

681 The valveless vertebral venous plexus runs the entire length of the vertebral column and has both external and internal components which

anastomose freely with each other as well as with lumbar, intercostal and pelvic veins. The internal plexus lies within the extradural space and is arranged in four longitudinal channels. The prostatic venous plexus is thought to communicate directly with this venous system, and thus explains the occurrence of early prostatic metastases in the vertebrae and skull.
[I:578; J:144]

682 Compression of the sacral plexus will cause sciatica and low back ache. If the dorsal rami are also affected then the erector spinae of the lumbosacral region may go into spasm.
[E:279; G:373]

683 The lateral part of the upper arm is supplied by the C5 dermatome. X-rays of the middle and lower cervical vertebrae, especially the C4/5 intervertebral space, might well produce a diagnosis.
[I:542; J:96]

684 This is the classic presentation of bilateral cervical ribs causing pressure on the T1 nerve roots. Sometimes these ribs can be seen to articulate with the first rib or may even simulate a lesion in the apex of the lung.
[E:63; G:17]

C Information answers

685 The pia mater closely invests the spinal cord. On each side thickenings are formed in it between the nerve roots—the denticulate ligaments. These pass laterally across the subarachnoid space to fuse with the arachnoid and dura mater. They assist the spinal cord's suspension in the centre of the meningeal sheath.
[A:992; E:828; H:83]

686 The pia mater, having covered the spinal cord throughout its length, continues as a thread from the apex of its termination, through the subarachnoid space to be attached to the coccyx inferiorly. This thread of pia is called the filum terminale.
[A:807; G:548; H:84]

687 The spinal cord terminates at the level of the lower border of L1 in the adult. The spinal theca terminates at the level of S2 and therefore the subarachnoid space ends at this level. Lumbar puncture is carried out between these two levels, usually at L4/5. In the infant, the spinal cord ends at a lower level than in the adult— around L3/4.
[A:806; D:354; E:822]

688 There are 31 pairs of spinal nerves subdivided as follows: cervical 8, thoracic 12, lumbar 5, sacral 5, coccygeal 1.
[A:1030; G:540]

689 The spinal cord runs in the vertebral canal surrounded by three membranes. The pia closely invests the cord; the dura and arachnoid are in apposition and lie close to the circumference of the vertebral canal. There is a space between arachnoid and pia—the subarachnoid space. This is filled with shock-absorbing fluid—the cerebrospinal fluid.
[A:992; G:548; H:84]

690 The dural sheath lies in the vertebral canal but is separated from its walls by the extradural space, which is filled with loose areolar tissue and fat. Embedded in this fascia is a plexus of veins, the internal vertebral venous plexus. The importance of the extradural space is that the spinal nerve roots traverse it and hence may be blocked by an injection of local anaesthetic in this region. Furthermore, the venous plexus may be damaged during a traumatic lumbar puncture with a resultant bloody tap.
[A:989; E:815]

691 The dura mater sends tubular lateral prolongations which surround each root of the spinal nerves. These prolongations eventually become continuous with the epineurium of the mixed spinal nerve as it passes through the intervertebral foramen. Although short in the upper region of the cord, the prolongations become longer inferiorly because of the increasing obliquity of nerve roots due to difference in growth between cord and spine.
[A:992; E:815; J:118]

C Applied answers

692 The contrast medium is within the subarachnoid space which extends along the spinal nerve roots, and consequently these are seen on normal x-rays as small lateral extensions.
[I:566; J:112]

693 During development, the vertebral column outgrows the spinal cord. In most adults the cord ends at the lower border of L1; that of the newborn infant extends slightly lower, to the third lumbar vertebra. In most infants, and even a few adults, a lumbar puncture performed at L2 may cause laceration of the spinal cord, with subsequent paralysis and sensory loss.
[E:822]

694 In a lateral view the anterior margin of the thecal sac has slight concavities due to the bulging of the annulus fibrosus of the normal intervertebral disc. These are normally checked—especially those of the lumbar region—for herniation, in patients with back pain and sciatica.
[I:566; J:118]

695 Particularly in the cervical region, the intervertebral foramen is relatively narrow to accommodate its spinal vessels and nerve. As the foramen is not capable of expansion due to its bony walls, compression—particularly of the nerve—can easily happen. This gives rise to root pains felt over the appropriate dermatomes.
[G:56; H:75]

696 With the patient sitting or lying in the fetal position, a lumbar puncture needle entering the back will pierce, in succession: skin, subcutaneous tissues, supraspinous and interspinous ligaments, and the ligamentum flavum if the needle is not absolutely midline. The elastic ligamentum flavum is felt as a definite resistance. The needle will then cross the epidural space containing the posterior intervertebral venous plexus and thence through the dura and arachnoid mater (spinal theca) to enter the

subarachnoid space. Here the needle tip will be bathed in CSF and lie amongst the lumbosacral nerve roots of the cauda equina.
[E:818]

4
Biographical notes on eponyms

ACHILLES
A mythical Greek warrior who was vulnerable only in the heel.
A' reflex – ankle jerk.
A' tendon – tendon of gastrocnemius and soleus (tendo calcaneus).

ALCOCK, Benjamin
1801–?. In 1849 was appointed Professor of Anatomy in Queen's College, Cork, but was called upon to resign in 1853 due to a dispute concerning the working of the Anatomy Acts. Went to USA in 1855, and was heard of no more!
A's canal – for the internal pudendal vessels in the ischiorectal fossa.

BAKER, William M.
1839–1896. An English surgeon.
B's cyst – a cyst of the bursa of the popliteal fossa.

BARTHOLIN, Caspar (Secundus)
1655–1738. Succeeded his father, Thomas Bartholin, as Professor of Medicine, Anatomy and Physics in Copenhagen.
B's ducts – sublingual ducts that open into the submandibular duct.
B's glands – greater vestibular glands.

BELL, Sir Charles
1774–1842. Surgeon, anatomist and artist. Founder of The Middlesex Hospital Medical School. Later Professor of Surgery, Edinburgh.
B's nerve – long thoracic nerve to serratus anterior.
B's palsy – facial nerve paralysis of unknown aetiology.

BIGELOW, Henry Jacob
1818–1890. Professor of Surgery at Harvard, USA.
B's ligament – the iliofemoral ligament, or the Y-shaped ligament of the hip joint.

BOCHDALEK, Vincent A.
1801–1883.   A Prague anatomist.
B's foramen – pleuroperitoneal canal.
B's gap – lumbocostal trigone.
B's gland – derived from primitive thyroglossal duct.

BOYDEN, Edward A.
1886–1978.   An American anatomist.
B's meal – fatty meal used to test gall bladder evacuation.
B's sphincter – the separate sphincter of the common bile duct proximal to the sphincter of Oddi.

BUCK, Gurdon
1807–1877.   A New York surgeon.
B's fascia – deep penile fascia.

CAMPER, Pieter
1722–1789.   Professor of Medicine, Anatomy, Surgery and Botany in Groningen, Holland, from 1763 to 1773.
C's fascia – fatty layer of the superficial fascia of the abdomen.

COLLES, Abraham
1773–1843.   Professor of Anatomy and Surgery in Dublin from 1804 to 1836.
C' fascia – perineal fascia and deep layer of the superficial fascia of the abdomen.
C' fracture – of the extremity of the radius.
C' ligament – reflected inguinal ligament.

COOPER, Sir Astley P.
1768–1841.   An English surgeon, Guy's Hospital, London.
C's fascia – cremasteric fascia.
Ligaments of C – fibrous tissue in the breast which accounts for dimpling of the skin in certain carcinomata. Suspensory ligaments.

CORTI, Alfonso
1822–1888.   An Italian anatomist.
Organ of C – Specialised cells within the cochlear duct, consisting of a basilar membrane supporting hair cells which rub against the tectorial membrane.

COWPER, William
1666–1709.   A London surgeon. FRS 1698.
C's glands – bulbourethral glands.

DOUGLAS, James
1675–1742. Scottish anatomist and 'man-midwife'
who lived in London. Physician to the Queen. FRS
1706.
Line of D – the arcuate line of the posterior layer of
the sheath of rectus abdominis.
Pouch of D – rectouterine peritoneal pouch.

DUPUYTREN, Guillaume
1777–1835. A French surgeon and pathologist.
D's contracture – fibrosis of palmar fascia causing
fixed flexion deformity usually of ring and little
fingers.

EDINGER, Ludwig
1855–1918. A German anatomist.
E–Westphal nucleus – midbrain group of cells forming part of the oculomotor nerve from which originate the preganglionic parasympathetic fibres to
the eye.

ERB, Wilhelm H.
1840–1921. A German neurologist.
E's palsy – damage to the upper trunk of the brachial
plexus.

EUSTACHIO (EUSTACHI or EUSTACHIUS), Barto-
lomeo
1520–1574. Professor of Anatomy in Rome, and Physician to the Pope.
Eustachian tube – the auditory tube (strictly, its cartilaginous part).
E valve – valve of the inferior vena cava.

FALLOPIUS (FALLOPIO), Gabriele
1523–1563. Professor of Anatomy and Surgery in
Padua.
F' canal – facial nerve canal.
Fallopian tube – uterine tube.

FRIEDREICH, Nikolas
1825–1882. A German neurologist.
F's ataxia – hereditary spinal ataxia.

FROMENT, Jules
1878–1946. Professor of Medicine, Lyons, France.
F's sign – seen in ulnar palsy when the distal phalanx
of thumb flexes whilst trying to hold a piece of
paper against the index finger. This due to adduc-

267

tor pollicis weakness permitting overaction of flexor pollicis longus.

GALEN, Claudius
c. 130–200. 2nd century physician and gatherer of medical information. Many of his erroneous ideas were regarded as gospel until the 15th and 16th centuries.
Great vein of G – internal cerebral vein.

GARTNER, Hermann Treschow
1785–1827. A Copenhagen anatomist.
G's canal or duct – the vestige of the mesonephric duct found in the broad ligament of the uterus and sometimes extending in the wall of the vagina to the vulva.

HESSELBACH, Franz K
1759–1816. A German surgeon.
H's fascia – cribriform fascia.
H's triangle – inguinal triangle.

HIGHMORE, Nathaniel
1613–1685. An English anatomist.
H's antrum – maxillary antrum.

HILTON, John
1804–1878. Surgeon at Guy's Hospital, London, from 1849 to 1871.
H's law – a nerve which crosses a joint, gives a branch to that joint.

HORNER, Johann F.
1831–1886. A Zürich ophthalmologist.
H's syndrome – facial and ophthalmic paresis, due to cervical sympathetic interruption.

HOUSTON, John
1802–1845. Lecturer in Surgery in Dublin, and Physician to the City Hospital.
Valves or folds of H – transverse rectal folds.

HUNT, James R.
1872–1937. An American neurologist.
H's syndrome – facial paralysis, otalgia, aural herpes due to geniculate ganglion herpes zoster.

HUNTER, John
1728–1793. A Scottish anatomist and surgeon who worked in London. Founder of the Hunterian Museum, now in the custody of the Royal College of Surgeons of England.
H's canal – adductor canal or subsartorial canal of the thigh.

KIESSELBACH, Wilhelm
1839–1902. German laryngologist.
K's area – anterior portion of nasal septum often site of epistaxis. (syn: Little's area.)

KILLIAN, Gustav
1860–1921. Berlin Professor of Otolaryngology.
K's bundle – lowest fibres of inferior constrictor of pharynx.
K's dehiscence – weakness between fibres of inferior pharyngeal constrictor.

KLUMPKE, Augusta Dejerine-
1859–1927. A French neurologist.
K's paralysis – paralysis of the intrinsic muscles of the hand, often due to birth injury.

LATARJET, Andre
1877–1947. A French anatomist.
L's nerve – a branch of the anterior vagus to the upper border of the pylorus and antrum of the stomach.

LOUIS, Antoine
1723–1792. A surgeon and physiologist of Paris whom American authorities cite as noting the 'angle' but this is not mentioned in his works.
Angle of L – the manubriosternal junction.

MACKENRODT, Alwin K.
1859–1925. Professor of Gynaecology in Berlin.
M's ligament – cardinal (lateral cervical) ligament of the uterus.

McBURNEY, Charles
1845–1914. A New York surgeon.
M's point – between $1\frac{1}{2}$ and 2 inches (3.8–5.0 cm) from the right anterior superior iliac spine upon a line to the umbilicus. The given site of maximum tenderness with appendicitis.

MECKEL, Johann Friedrich
1714–1774. Professor of Anatomy, Botany and Gynaecology in Berlin.
M's space/cave – the trigeminal cavum. The subarachnoid space around cranial nerve V as it lies in the middle cranial fossa.

MECKEL, Johann Friedrich the younger
1781–1833. Grandson of the preceding. A German comparative anatomist and embryologist.
M's cartilage – the cartilage of the first brachial arch.
M's diverticulum – a diverticulum of the ileum; a persistent proximal part of the vitellointestinal duct.

MEIBOMIUS (MEIBOM), Hendrik
1638–1700. Professor of Medicine at Helmstadt and later Professor of Poetic Art.
Meibomian cyst – chalazion due to infection of a tarsal gland.
M' gland – tarsal gland.

MONTGOMERY, William F.
1797–1859. Professor of Midwifery in Dublin.
M's tubercle – elevated reddish areolar glands easily seen in pregnancy.

MORGAGNI, Giovanni Battista
1682–1771. A Padua anatomist and pathologist.
Appendix or hydatid of M – appendix testis or vesicular appendix of epoöphoron.
Columns of M – anal columns.
Foramen of M – foramen caecum of the tongue.
Lacunae/Fossa of M – fossa navicularis.

MÜLLER, Heinrich
1820–1864. A German anatomist.
M's muscle – superior tarsal muscle of the eyelids, or circular fibres of the iris.

MÜLLER, Johannes Peter
1801–1858. Professor of Anatomy and Physiology in Berlin.
M's duct – primordial female genital duct—the paramesonephric duct.

ODDI, Ruggero
1864–1913. An Italian physician.
Sphincter of O – sphincteric muscle fibres around the termination of the bile duct and main pancreatic duct.

PAGET, Sir James
1814–1899. An English surgeon.
P's disease of nipple – malignant change in the skin surrounding the nipple.

PANCOAST, Henry Khunrath
1875–1939. Professor of Radiology in Pennsylvania, USA.
P's syndrome – apical carcinoma of lung associated with Horner's syndrome, brachial plexus palsy, pain down the arm and distension of neck veins.

PETIT, Jean Louis
1674–1750. A Paris surgeon.
P's triangle – lumbar triangle.

PEYER, Johan Konrad
1653–1712. Professor of Logic, Rhetoric and Medicine in Schaffhausen, Switzerland.
P's patches – aggregated lymphoid follicles in the lower ileum.

PFANNENSTIEL, Hermann Johann
1862–1909.
P's incision – transverse suprapubic incision used for pelvic surgery.

POTT, Percival
1713–1788. An English surgeon.
P's disease – tuberculosis of the spine.
P's fracture – ankle fractures involving the malleoli and ligaments.

POUPART, François
1661–1709. Surgeon to the Hotel Dieu, Paris.
P's ligament – inguinal ligament.

RAYNAUD, Maurice
1834–1881. A Parisian physician.
R's disease – peripheral vascular disturbance consisting of spasmodic contractions of the digital arteries.

REISSNER, Ernst
1824–1878. A German anatomist.
R's membrane – vestibular membrane of the inner ear, dividing scala vestibuli and scala media.

RIEDEL, Bernhard M. C. L.
1846–1916.   A German surgeon.
R's lobe – a tongue-like extension of the right lobe of
the liver.

SANTORINI, Giovanni D.
1681–1737.   An Italian anatomist.
Cartilage of S – corniculate cartilage.
Duct of S – accessory pancreatic duct.

SCARPA, Antonio
1747–1832.   A Venetian anatomist, orthopaedist and
ophthalmologist.
S's fascia – deep layer of the superficial fascia of the
lower abdomen.
S's nerve – nasopalatine nerve.
S's triangle – femoral triangle.

SCHLEMM, Friedrich S.
1795–1858.   A German anatomist.
Canal of S – venous sinus of the sclera found at the
corneoscleral junction.

SIBSON, Francis
1814–1876.   An English anatomist.
S's fascia – the suprapleural membrane.

SPIGELIUS, Adrian (van der Speighel)
1578–1625.   A Belgian anatomist in Padua.
Spigelian hernia – herniation along the linea semilunaris of the abdomen.
S' lobe – caudate lobe of liver.

STENSEN, Niels or Nicholaus
1638–1686.   Danish anatomist, who later became a
minister and a bishop.
S's duct – duct of the parotid gland lying across
masseter muscle.

TENON, Jacques René
1724–1816.   Professor of Pathology in the Academy
of Sciences, Paris, and Chief Surgeon at the Sal-
petrier.
T's capsule or fascia – the fascial sheath of the eyeball.

THEBESIUS, Adam C.
1686–1732.   A German physician.
T' valve – valve of the coronary sinus.

Thebesian veins – small veins draining directly into the cardiac chambers.

TRENDELENBURG, Freidrich
1844–1924. A German surgeon.
T position – operating position with head down and pelvis elevated, as used in the treatment of shock.
T sign – dipping of the pelvis in congenital hip dislocation.

VATER, Abraham
1684–1751. Professor of Anatomy, Botany, Pathology and Therapeutics in Wittenberg, Germany.
Ampulla of V – hepatopancreatic ampulla.

VIDIUS (Guido Guidi)
1500–1569. Italian anatomist and physician to Francis I of France; from 1548, Professor of Medicine at Pisa.
V canal – pterygoid canal.
V nerve – nerve of pterygoid canal.

VOLKMANN, Richard von
1830–1889. German Professor of Surgery.
V's contracture – tissue loss, especially muscular, due to ischaemia.
V's splint – guttered splint for lower extremity fractures.

WALDEYER, Heinrich W. G. von
1836–1921. Professor of Pathological Anatomy in Breslau, and later in Berlin.
W's ring – lymphatic ring in the pharynx.

WESTPHAL, Karl F. O.
1833–1890. A German neurologist.
Edinger–W nucleus – group of cells in midbrain forming part of the oculomotor nerve from which preganglionic parasympathetic fibres to the eye are derived.

WHARTON, Thomas
1614–1673. An English anatomist.
W's duct – main submandibular duct opening at the frenulum of the tongue.
W's jelly – connective tissue (mucous) of umbilical cord.

WINSLOW, Jacob Benignus
1669–1760.   A Danish anatomist who, at the age of 74, was appointed Professor of Anatomy, Physics and Surgery in Paris.
Foramen of W – epiploic foramen.
Ligament of W – oblique popliteal ligament.
Pancreas of W – uncinate process of the pancreas.

WIRSUNG, Johann G.
1600–1643.   A German anatomist in Padua.
W's duct – the main pancreatic duct.

WOLFF, Kaspar Friedrich
1733–1794.   Professor of Anatomy and Physiology in St Petersburg. One of the founders of modern embryology.
W'ian duct – mesonephric duct.
W'ian body – mesonephros.